Getting into GP Training

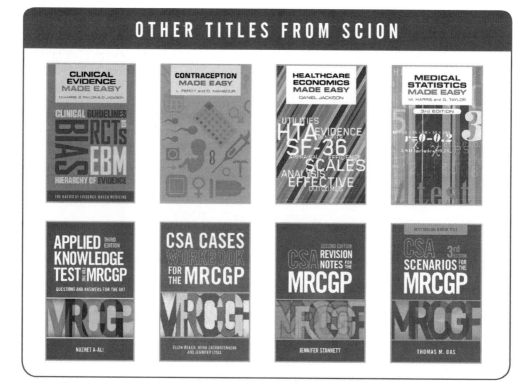

Getting into GP Training

A complete guide to Stages 1, 2, 3 and 4

Ciarán Conway

BMedSci (Hons), BMBS, DRCOG, PGCert
ST1 in General Practice, Bath, UK

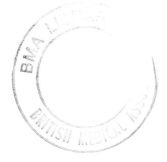

Scion

© **Scion Publishing Limited, 2016**

First published 2016

A CIP catalogue record for this book is available from the British Library.

ISBN 978 1 904842 25 5

Scion Publishing Limited

The Old Hayloft, Vantage Business Park, Bloxham Road, Banbury OX16 9UX, UK
www.scionpublishing.com

Important Note from the Publisher

The information contained within this book was obtained by Scion Publishing Ltd from sources believed by us to be reliable. However, while every effort has been made to ensure its accuracy, no responsibility for loss or injury whatsoever occasioned to any person acting or refraining from action as a result of information contained herein can be accepted by the authors or publishers.

Readers are reminded that medicine is a constantly evolving science and while the authors and publishers have ensured that all dosages, applications and practices are based on current indications, there may be specific practices which differ between communities. You should always follow the guidelines laid down by the manufacturers of specific products and the relevant authorities in the country in which you are practising.

Although every effort has been made to ensure that all owners of copyright material have been acknowledged in this publication, we would be pleased to acknowledge in subsequent reprints or editions any omissions brought to our attention.

Registered names, trademarks, etc. used in this book, even when not marked as such, are not to be considered unprotected by law.

Typeset by Phoenix Photosetting, Chatham, Kent, UK
Printed in the UK

To
Suzy, Mum and Dad
for their endless support

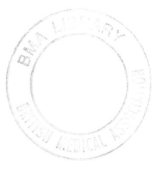

Contents

Preface

This book has been written for anyone who is thinking about applying for specialty training in General Practice (GP) in the UK and Northern Ireland. Its purpose is to guide the reader through the tortuous application process from start to finish. Included within are individual chapters on each of the application stages, together with full practice papers for Stages 2 and 3.

I genuinely hope that this book helps you in the first step on your journey to becoming a GP.

Ciarán Conway
August 2015

Acknowledgements

I would like to thank all of those who have helped in the creation of this book by reviewing drafts and offering support in a variety of forms. In particular I would like to thank: Dr Christopher Phillips, Dr Christopher White, Dr James Smith, Mr David Thurtle, Dr Samuel Walker, Dr James O'Connor, Dr Sarina Patel, Dr Thomas Rutter and Mr Benedict Conway.

List of abbreviations

ABG	Arterial blood gas
A&E	Accident and Emergency Department
ACE	Angiotensin-converting enzyme
ACF	Academic Clinical Fellowship
ALS	Advanced life support
BCC	Basal cell carcinoma
BCG	Bacillus Calmette–Guérin vaccine
BNF	*British National Formulary*
bpm	Beats per minute
BPPV	Benign paroxysmal positional vertigo
BTS	British Thoracic Society
BV	Bacterial vaginosis
COCP	Combined oral contraceptive pill
COPD	Chronic obstructive pulmonary disease
CRB	Criminal Records Bureau
CPR	Cardiopulmonary resuscitation
CT	Computerised tomography
DBS	Disclosure and Barring Service
DKA	Diabetic ketoacidosis
DOPs	Directly observed procedures
DPP-4	Dipeptidyl peptidase-4
DVLA	Driver and Vehicle Licensing Agency
EBV	Epstein–Barr virus
ECG	Electrocardiogram
EMQ	Extended Matching Question
ENT	Ear, nose and throat

ERCP	Endoscopic retrograde cholangiopancreatography
FPAS	Foundation Programme application system
FY1	Foundation Year One Doctor
FY2	Foundation Year Two Doctor
GCS	Glasgow Coma Scale
GMC	General Medical Council
GP	General practice
GPVTS	General Practice Vocational Training Scheme
HbA1c	Glycated haemoglobin
HIV	Human immunodeficiency virus
HPA	Health Protection Agency
HPV	Human papillomavirus
HRT	Hormone replacement therapy
I.M.	Intramuscular
I.V.	Intravenous
ICE	Ideas, concerns, expectations
IELTS	International English Language Testing System
IgE	Immunoglobulin E
INR	International normalised ratio
JVP	Jugular venous pressure
LABA	Long-acting beta agonist
LETB	Local Education and Training Board
M.I.	Myocardial infarction
mcg	Micrograms
MCQ	Multiple Choice Question
mg	Milligrams
mmol/L	Millimoles per litre
N.I. Number	National Insurance Number
NICE	National Institute for Health and Care Excellence
NRO	National Recruitment Office
NSAID	Non-steroidal anti-inflammatory drug
OSCE	Objective Structured Clinical Examination
P.O.	*Per os* (by mouth)
PALS	Patient Advice Liaison Service
PEF	Peak expiratory flow
POP	Progesterone-only pill

RCGP	Royal College of General Practitioners
SAU	Surgical Assessment Unit
SHO	Senior House Officer
SJT	Situational Judgment Test
TIA	Transient ischaemic attack
UK & NI	United Kingdom and Northern Ireland
UK MEC	The United Kingdom Medical Eligibility Criteria

Chapter 1
Introduction to the GP application process

*"The fight is won or lost far away from witnesses –
behind the lines, in the gym, and out there on the road,
long before I dance under those lights."*

Muhammad Ali

It might seem strange to start a book about the GP application process with a quote from one of the greatest boxers of all time, but this quote encapsulates the attitude you should adopt in order to get your dream GP training post. Your success in this application process will be almost entirely decided by what you do between now and when you sit the Stage 2 and Stage 3 exams – long before you sit down to take them.

There has been recent press coverage highlighting a "recruitment crisis" in general practice. The severity of this issue has prompted discussions at the highest levels of government and has led the Royal College of General Practitioners (RCGP) to launch a campaign to improve the image of life as a GP. This may lead you to think that gaining a training post is therefore a straightforward process. It is not.

Even a cursory look at the competition ratios for the last five years (*Appendix*) will reveal that, in most deaneries, competition remains fierce and that in deaneries such as London there are more than three applicants for each training post. In short, while overall recruitment may be down, competition for places in the more popular deaneries remains as strong as ever.

The GP application is a prolonged process. It starts in November and can continue right through to the end of the spring and therefore it is advantageous to have a good idea of how the overall process works. This will help you focus on the various aspects of the application appropriately and will allow you to maximise your chances of getting your first choice training post. The whole process can be split into four stages (*Figure 1.1*).

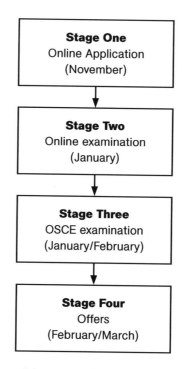

Figure 1.1 – Overview of the stages of application and approximate timing

Stage 1   This consists of completing the online application form available via the new Oriel recruitment system *(Appendix)*. The purpose of the form is to ensure that you are eligible to apply for GP training. It is available in early November (the exact date changes from year to year) and the deadline for its submission is usually the first week of December.

Stage 2   Stage 2 is an online assessment which takes place in the first weeks of January. It is a timed examination which consists of questions which test candidates' clinical problem solving skills and their ability to manage a series of professional dilemmas.

Stage 3   Stage 3 is an OSCE-style examination which tests candidates' communication skills. These exams take place at a variety of locations in January and into February.

Stage 4   Stage 4 refers to the offers process. Hopefully this stage will involve you being offered, and accepting, your first choice training post. However, this is not guaranteed and therefore this stage may involve applying through the clearing process for jobs elsewhere in the country.

You can be reassured that the majority of candidates will progress smoothly through the process and get a training post at the end. A small minority will not reach the point of being offered a training post; we will discuss how to avoid this throughout the book. The chapters that follow address each of the application stages individually and outline what to expect and how to avoid common pitfalls; they also provide practice examples of the types of assessments you will face.

> ## REMEMBER!
>
> The exact dates and deadlines of the application process change annually. Therefore it is crucial to keep a close eye on the GP National Recruitment Office (NRO) website so that you know exactly when the deadline is for each stage.

Chapter 2
Stage 1 explained

Stage 1 involves the completion of an online application form which is available via the Oriel recruitment portal or via a link on the GP National Recruitment Office (NRO) website *(Appendix)*. It should, in theory, be a straightforward process. However, it is a long form with many aspects to it, so it is worth having an idea of what is expected. Additionally, many prospective GP trainees have had years out of formal training or have done other training posts prior to applying so it can be difficult to know exactly how to fit your personal experiences into the format required.

Typically the online application form becomes available in early November and is accessible for around one month, closing in early December. The exact dates vary each year and therefore it is crucial to keep an eye on the NRO website so that you don't miss the deadlines.

It is important to remember that the purpose of the Stage 1 application form is to ensure that you are eligible to apply for GP training in the UK & NI and that you meet the basic levels of training required to progress to the Stage 2 assessment. It is <u>not</u> used to rank you in any way. It is crucial to ensure that you fill in the form correctly and completely to ensure progression to the next stage. **Incomplete forms and late entries will not be accepted**.

What's on the form?

As mentioned above, the purpose of the form is to establish your eligibility for GP training and therefore the first part asks if you have ever been removed or resigned from a GP training post. For most candidates this is a straightforward question with a straightforward answer. If this question does apply to you then you will need to seek individual guidance from the NRO as to whether you are still eligible to apply.

The opening section continues with a selection of questions about your personal information (Name, Address, N.I Number etc.). Following this, you're required to detail any current training number you may have. Being in a training post for an alternative specialty won't count for or against you but you must be honest if asked to provide further details.

The next section covers "less than full-time training" and "deferred entry" into a GP training programme. This part of the application could apply to you for a multitude of reasons such as if you are pregnant at the time of applying, have an illness, or another extenuating circumstance. If you are unsure if you qualify then you should seek guidance from the NRO before submitting your completed form.

The form then addresses the issue of whether or not you have a current and valid licence to practise in the UK. For the vast majority of those applying for training, this is a simple question to answer. However, there are a growing group who do not have a full UK licence at the time of applying and therefore need to explain why this is. For example, if you are working in New Zealand at the time of applying and have elected not to pay to keep your full licence in the UK then you would click "No" and then offer this explanation. So long as you have a legitimate explanation for why you haven't got a full licence then this question should not cause any issues.

For most candidates whose primary medical degree was in the UK, or taught in English, the next section regarding English language skills should be straightforward. If, however, your degree wasn't taught in English then you will need to prove that your English is of a sufficient standard. This will usually be by proving that you have acquired the appropriate level of achievement in the IELTS (International English Language Testing System). Candidates must also prove their nationality and, for overseas candidates, that they are eligible to practise in the UK.

There are then a series of questions regarding fitness to practise and pending, current, or previous criminal convictions. It's important that you are honest about these. If you are unsure about how to fill this part of the form in correctly then you should seek advice from the NRO directly.

You must then provide the contact details of three referees (and their secretaries). One of these referees must be your most recent (or current) clinical supervisor. These people won't be contacted until much later in the process but you must ask them personally if they would be happy to be a referee before you provide their details.

The majority of junior doctors applying for GPVTS (General Practice Vocational Training Scheme) will have completed, or be undertaking, a UK Foundation Programme and therefore can provide their "Foundation Achievement of Competency Document" (FACD 5.2) as proof of achievement of the foundation competencies. However, if this does not apply to you then you will need to find alternative evidence to prove that you have met the basic standards required.

Candidates must then provide details of their primary medical qualification followed by details of all posts since qualification. It's important to enter the dates of these posts accurately and to provide an explanation for any gaps in employment which are greater than four weeks.

GP trainees are required to do domiciliary visits and therefore candidates are asked to confirm that they have a UK driving licence. If you do not hold a full licence you will be asked to confirm that you will be willing to provide alternative means of transport.

For those candidates applying from abroad there is then a chance to state where you would like to sit the Stage 2 assessment as the UK NRO now offer exam centres outside of the UK & NI.

You are then asked to rank the Local Education Training Board (LETB) Deaneries in preference order. As of 2014/15 there are 15 possible deaneries (*Figure 2.1*); the number of places and the competition for each deanery varies from year to year (*Appendix*). Candidates must rank a minimum of six deaneries, although it is possible to rank them all. Should you not wish to be considered for a particular deanery then there is an option to put an "X" next to such deaneries. More information on how your ranking of these deaneries will impact on where you get a post can be found in *Chapter 5 – Stage 3 Explained*.

UK and Northern Ireland Deaneries
Health Education Thames Valley
London Recruitment
Health Education East of England
Health Education East Midlands
Health Education Kent, Surrey and Sussex
Health Education Yorkshire and the Humber
Defence Medical Services
Health Education North East
Health Education North West
Health Education South West
Health Education Wessex
Health Education West Midlands
Northern Ireland
Scotland
Wales

Figure 2.1 – List of the UK and Northern Ireland LETB Deaneries

The last part of the form asks for some details about equality and diversity and the final page of the form is a declaration which must be acknowledged prior to submission.

Academic Clinical Fellowships

Each year there are a limited number of Academic Clinical Fellowships (ACFs) available for general practice. The ACF posts are 4 year posts which focus on the academic aspects of general practice. They have benefits such as extra study budget, specific time set aside for academic pursuits such as projects and research, and the allocation of an academic supervisor. The number of posts available varies every year and not all deaneries offer them. They are highly competitive posts and can be applied for in parallel to the normal GPVTS application via the Oriel recruitment system. Further details are available from both the NRO website and the individual websites of the deaneries offering these posts. If you choose to apply for one of these posts you will need to provide an extra referee who can vouch for your academic experiences.

Top tips for Stage 1

- Do not leave this form until the last minute as it takes a long time to complete and mistakes will easily be made if you are rushing.

- Although you can save your entry and come back to it, it is better to set aside a quiet evening and do it in one go.

- Have all of your documents with you when you sit down to do it as it will save you time.

- For individual dates of your previous jobs, consult your NHS e-portfolio (if you have one) as they are recorded there and this will save time.

- Ask your referees if they are happy to provide a reference before submitting their details.

- If you are unsure how to complete any part of the form then consult the NRO website, or failing that email the NRO – it's important to fill this form in correctly to ensure progression to Stage 2.

- Before submitting the form check it extensively for any mistakes.

- Do not wait until the final day to submit the form.

REMEMBER!

You cannot progress to Stage 2 if the form is incorrectly completed. So take time to ensure there are no errors!
If you have any queries or concerns when filling in the form consult the NRO website or contact the NRO directly.

Chapter 3
Stage 2 explained

After successfully proving eligibility during Stage 1, candidates are invited to Stage 2. You cannot book a Stage 2 exam place until you receive an email giving you permission to do so. It is therefore important to keep a close eye on your emails after you have submitted your Stage 1 application as the Stage 2 exam places are allocated on a first come first served basis. If you want to sit the Stage 2 exam in your local exam centre at a time to suit you then you need to act quickly once you have received your invitation to book a place.

Stage 2 is an online examination which takes place throughout the country over several days in the first weeks of January. The exam takes place at Pearson Vue test centres throughout the UK, Northern Ireland and a limited number of locations outside of Europe. All of the exams are standardised to ensure that the level of questions are similar. The NRO spends a huge amount of time ensuring the fairness of their assessments and therefore it shouldn't matter which day or time that you sit your exam.

The online format of the exam is very intuitive and self-explanatory, but if you would feel happier by using the software prior to the day you can access an online tutorial via the Pearson Vue website (*Appendix*). This guides users through a series of screens and familiarises you with the controls and format.

It is important to remember that this exam is not a "pass or fail" assessment. Instead, your success is entirely dependent on how you perform relative to your peers. A very small minority of candidates with the lowest scores in Stage 2 will be deemed to have shown insufficient evidence of the level of knowledge required to progress further and their application will end at this point.

For candidates whose applications cease at this point there is an opportunity to reapply during the second round of applications. The second round of applications (often called "Round one re-advert") arises when the NRO offer candidates the opportunity to apply for unfilled training posts, in undersubscribed deaneries. This round is typically open to applications in March and is available both to candidates who have not been successful in the first round of applications and to new candidates. The application process remains the same and candidates must successfully sit the Stage 2 and 3 assessments in order to be offered a training post.

Details of how your performance in Stage 2 leads to allocation of a deanery are discussed in *Chapter 5 – Stage 3 Explained.*

On the day of the exam arrive in plenty of time. There are lots of invigilators present during the exam who will help you with any technical or personal issues that could arise. Be sure to thoroughly read the instructions sent to you in your confirmation email as there are specific details regarding what to take with you on the day (including what identification is required to sit the exam).

The Stage 2 exam is divided into two sections: a Professional Dilemma section and a Clinical Problem Solving section.

The Professional Dilemma section

This section lasts for 110 minutes and contains approximately 55 questions. Professional Dilemma questions examine a candidate's ability to act appropriately to a fictional scenario. The level at which your answer is compared to is that which a Foundation Year Two Doctor (FY2) would be expected to achieve. The questions take two main forms; 'ranking questions' and 'multiple best answer questions'. Both types are discussed in more detail below. They are similar in that both question types begin with a scenario followed by a list of options. By their very nature these questions are very subjective and there may not be right or wrong answers, so it is important to consider the questions calmly and not get frustrated.

The most abundant question format is the 'ranking question'. These offer the candidate five different options which must be ranked in order of appropriateness (or in the order in which you would do them). All of the options may be appropriate but you must rank them in the most appropriate order. There are, however, answers which are more right than others and these answers are the ones that most closely match the order set out by the examiners; you can still gain credit for an order which is close to that of the exact answer.

The second question format used in this part of the exam is the 'multiple best answer question' in which the candidate must choose one, two or three correct answers from a selection of different options. The best way to illustrate the two question types is with worked examples *(Sample Questions 3.1 and 3.2).*

Practice Scenario 1: Ranking Question

You are an FY2 doctor on a busy medical ward. You are taking urgent blood samples from a patient when you are distracted by an emergency on the ward. In order to help with the unfolding incident you put the blood samples in your pocket. Several hours later you realise that you have forgotten to send the samples to the laboratory. Unfortunately, the blood samples have clotted while in your pocket and are now unusable. Rank the following in the order you would do them:

A. Fill in an incident form.

B. Apologise to the patient for your error.

C. Do nothing.

D. Retake the blood tests.

E. Inform your supervising consultant of your error.

Sample Question 3.1 – Practice Scenario 1: Ranking Question

This question *(Sample Question 3.1)* is fairly typical of a Stage 2 exam question. With these questions it is usually (although not always) easy to identify the most and least appropriate answers. Here the most appropriate answer is "B. *Apologise to the patient for your error*". The GMC has issued guidance for adverse events in which it states that you should be open and honest with patients when things go wrong. The least appropriate answer is clearly "C. *Do nothing*" which would show a complete lack of insight into the consequence of this error. Answer "D. *Retake the blood tests*" is the second most appropriate answer. You ought to let your supervising consultant know what has happened (option E). These were urgent blood samples and the delay in getting the results may impact on the patient's care. You should then complete an incident form (option A). With all of this in mind the correct order would be B, D, E, A, C. As we have discussed previously the very nature of these questions means that the answers are subjective. Don't worry if you did not get the order exactly right, you can still get credit for getting the order partially correct.

Practice Scenario 2: Multiple Best Answer Question

You are an FY2 doctor and during your General Practice placement you see a 40-year-old married man who admits to having had unprotected sexual intercourse with a sex worker during a recent business trip. He wishes to be investigated for sexually transmitted infections as he has noticed some penile discharge recently. He has opted not to tell his wife, who is also a patient of yours, and has continued to have unprotected sexual intercourse with her.

Choose the **three** most appropriate actions:

A. Call the patient's wife to inform her of his recent behaviour.

B. Advise the patient that he is putting his wife at risk by continuing to have unprotected sex with her.

C. Refuse to treat the patient.

D. Take a sexual history from the patient's wife when she next attends your clinic.

E. Take a full history and examination of the patient.

F. Inform the patient that you find his behaviour appalling.

G. Offer the patient appropriate investigations and treatment.

H. Tell your colleagues about the case at your next coffee break.

Sample Question 3.2 – Practice Scenario 2: Multiple Best Answer Question

Multiple best answer questions (*Sample Question 3.2*) require you to select a certain number of responses which are more appropriate than the rest. The crucial thing to remember with these questions is to select the correct number of answers as these can vary with some questions asking for two, three or more correct answers. A silly way to drop marks would be by not selecting the correct number of responses. The multiple best answer question above is a typical Stage 2 question which does not test any specific medical knowledge but instead focuses on the practice of medicine. The question is really about confidentiality between you and the patient and therefore the correct answers here are B, E and G. While it may be tempting to tell his wife in order to protect her (she is after all your patient too) or to gossip to your colleagues about the case, this would actually be a breach of confidentiality. Equally, it would be inappropriate to inform the patient that you find his behaviour appalling, or not to treat him.

Those candidates who graduated from a UK-based medical school after 2011 will be fairly familiar with both formats of questions as they will have taken part in the Foundation Programme Application System (FPAS) in which these styles of questions are used. Their subjective nature makes them difficult to prepare for but this does not mean that you cannot improve your technique. Some useful things to do in order to prepare for the Professional Dilemma section of the Stage 2 exam are:

- Read the GP National Personal Specification which is useful in identifying the qualities that the questions will be examining (*Appendix*)

- Read the GMC's "Good Medical Practice." This guide covers a vast array of common scenarios faced by doctors and how the GMC would expect their members to act. (*Appendix*)

- Try to use your everyday job as practice by imagining scenarios based around things you see and do at work

- Practise the scenarios in the Stage 2 practice paper (*Chapter 4*)

- Speak to people who have done the Stage 2 exam in previous years

It is more than likely that you will leave the exam on the day unsure how well you did in this section. Unfortunately that is the nature of the question format. However, by practising this question format extensively you will at least be in a better position from which to tackle each scenario.

The Clinical Problem Solving section

This section lasts for 75 minutes and contains approximately 100 questions. This part of the exam tests your medical knowledge and therefore, due to its objectivity, is easier to prepare for than the Professional Dilemmas section. The clinical questions are set at a level of knowledge that would be expected from an FY2. This is an important thing to bear in mind when practising for this exam. Many people incorrectly believe that this exam will be easy and straightforward and some candidates fail to revise appropriately. In a true reflection of life as a GP this exam focuses on breadth, and not depth, of knowledge. This key differentiation is where many candidates fall down. There is no use being able to cite the pharmacology of a novel cancer therapy which is used exclusively in tertiary centre management if you know nothing about the first line treatment of asthma for example. It is worth keeping this in mind throughout your revision. There are a wide range of topics that the exam could potentially cover (*Figure 3.1*).

This list is by no means exhaustive but does give you an idea of the types of things that could be included in the exam. It is worth going through the list and deciding which areas you are least confident in and start by revising these topics. The exam tends to sample something from almost each area, so a broad knowledge base is important.

Potential topic areas include (but are not limited to):

- Pharmacology
- Obstetrics and Gynaecology
- Urology and Sexual Health
- Psychiatry
- Orthopaedics and Rheumatology
- Ophthalmology
- Otorhinolaryngology (ENT)
- Endocrinology
- Surgery and Breast Disease
- Genetics
- Cardiovascular medicine
- Chest medicine
- Neurology
- Gastroenterology
- Renal
- Dermatology
- Paediatrics
- Haematology and Infectious Diseases
- Acute/Emergency Medicine

Figure 3.1 – A list of potential subjects for Stage Two – Clinical Problem Solving questions.

The questions in this part of the exam mostly take the form of a mixture of Multiple Choice Questions (MCQs) and Extended Matching Questions (EMQs). Both types of questions are commonly used in both undergraduate and postgraduate medical exams and therefore will be familiar to most readers; however an example of each question format is provided below for your benefit *(Sample Questions 3.4 and 3.5).*

MCQ Example

A 52-year-old man presents acutely with lethargy and a painful arthritis affecting his left knee and some of the small joints of his hands and feet. His only past medical history of note is a recent bout of severe gastroenteritis a month ago while on a business trip in the Far East. Which of the following is the most likely diagnosis?

A. Osteoarthritis
B. Ankylosing spondylitis
C. Reactive arthritis
D. Rheumatoid arthritis
E. Whipple's disease

Sample Question 3.4 – MCQ Example

Sample Question 3.4 is quite typical of those in the Clinical Problem Solving section of the Stage 2 exam. The correct answer here is "C. Reactive arthritis". Reactive arthritis is an asymmetrical arthritis which often follows a gastro-intestinal or genitourinary infection (typically 2–6 weeks later) and affects one or more joints. Note that the question asks for "the most likely diagnosis" – this is important as with many of these questions there may be more than one answer that could be correct in practice but may not be "the most likely" of the options.

EMQ Example

Regarding the breast:
A. Paget's disease of the breast
B. Mastalgia
C. Gynaecomastia
D. Fibroadenoma
E. Lipoma
F. Sebaceous cyst
G. Breast cancer
H. Breast abscess

For each of the following scenarios choose the most likely diagnosis or symptom. Each answer may be used once, more than once, or not at all.

1. A 75-year-old man presents because he has developed increased breast tissue over the last few months. He finds this uncomfortable and he is embarrassed by it. His only past medical history is of prostate cancer for which he is being treated with hormonal therapy.

2. A 50-year-old patient presents because she has noticed that her right nipple appears to have developed an area of eczema-like change. On examination there is a well demarcated erythematous patch overlying the right nipple which is distorting the nipple architecture.

3. A 30-year-old patient who is currently breast feeding develops a painful erythematous region of the right breast over a number of days. On examination she is pyrexial.

Sample Question 3.5 – EMQ Example

The correct answers here (*Sample Question 3.5*) are C, A and H. It is important with the extended matching questions to note that often the question will stipulate that the answers can be used "once, more than once, or not at all." In the actual exam the EMQs are spread over a number of pages with all the available answers and only one question at a time visible, but here they are presented with all three questions visible.

Keep in mind when you are revising that a variety of different areas will be examined. The questions in the Clinical Problem Solving section include diagnosis, investigation, treatment and management and therefore a good broad base of knowledge is required to do well in this part of the exam.

REMEMBER!

- Keep an eye out for the invitation email and book your exam as soon as possible to ensure you sit the exam when and where you want.
- Take the exam seriously by revising topics that you aren't confident with.
- Practise, Practise, Practise.
- The exam focuses on breadth, and not depth, of knowledge.
- Try the full Stage 2 practice papers available in *Chapter 4*.
- Read the instructions sent to you about Stage 2 so that you know exactly what to take with you on the day.

Chapter 4
Stage 2 practice paper

This exam is made up of two papers. The first contains 55 Professional Dilemma questions for which you are allowed 110 minutes (2 minutes per question on average). The second is made up of 100 Clinical Problem Solving questions for which you are allowed 75 minutes (45 seconds per question).

You may not want to do the whole paper in one go, but it is good practice to keep to the time schedule. So you might want to attempt 10 Professional Dilemma questions in 20 minutes for example.

Answers and explanations can be found in the answer section at the end of the book.

Professional Dilemma questions

55 Questions

Time Limit: 110 minutes

1. You are an FY2 doctor on the pre-operative ward round with your registrar who is consenting patients for this morning's theatre list. You notice that your registrar is behaving oddly and on closer inspection smells of alcohol. You strongly suspect that he is drunk. Rank the following actions in the most appropriate order.

    A. Speak to your registrar directly about your concerns.
    B. Contact the General Medical Council (GMC).
    C. Speak to your consultant about your concerns.
    D. Take no action.
    E. Take advice on how to act from your medical defence body.

2. The son of a patient under your care phones the ward from Brazil for an update on his mother's condition. Unfortunately, his mother has been unconscious since admission due to severe sepsis and you update him accordingly. Over the next week the patient improves substantially and regains consciousness. She expressly states that no information about her condition should be given to her son from whom she has been estranged for many years. Rank the following in order of appropriateness.

    A. Don't tell the patient that you have told her son details of her condition.
    B. Apologise to the patient and explain what has happened.
    C. Inform your supervising consultant of the details of the incident.
    D. Ensure that you do not tell the son any more information if he should phone again.
    E. Make a reflective entry in your e-portfolio about the incident.

3. You are an A&E FY2 doctor. A patient presents to the minors unit with an injured ankle. It transpires that the patient is one of the senior nurses from the hospital's orthopaedic ward and she believes that she has fractured her ankle while dancing at a party last night. She is demanding an X-ray. You thoroughly examine her and feel that her ankle doesn't meet any clinical criteria for an X-ray. Rank the following in order of appropriateness.

    A. Offer the patient verbal and written advice about ankle sprains.

    B. Order an X-ray.

    C. Explain your clinical findings to the patient and explain your rationale for not ordering an X-ray.

    D. Explore the patient's ideas and concerns about her ankle injury.

    E. Advise the patient to return or see her GP if symptoms do not improve.

4. While working on a general medical ward you have finished most of your ward jobs and are able to find a spare half an hour to work on a job application that is due in this evening. A staff nurse asks you if you could help her by countersigning a bag of fluids which she is about to give to a patient. She cannot find anyone else to ask because the ward is so short staffed. Rank the following options in order of appropriateness.

    A. Refuse to help.

    B. Agree to help the nurse and countersign the fluids appropriately.

    C. Fill out an incident form regarding the staffing level on the ward.

    D. Explain to the nurse that you can't help as your job application is due in this evening and you need every available minute to complete it.

    E. Make a reflective entry in your e-portfolio about time management.

5. You are the FY2 on a medical consultant ward round. The consultant has seen a patient and formulated a management plan and you have clearly documented this in the notes. You return to the patient after the ward round to complete the tasks and find two of the nursing staff loudly criticising the plan at the nurses' station. Rank the following options in order of appropriateness.

    A. Report both nurses to their professional governing body for misconduct.

    B. Tell the nurses it is not your plan but the consultant's and that you agree that the plan is poor.

    C. Inform the ward sister about their behaviour.

    D. Explain the reasoning behind the plan to the nurses.

    E. Explore their reasons for the criticism.

6. You are a general surgery FY2 doctor. During the pre-operative ward round your registrar asks you to consent the last patient on the list for him while he goes to theatre to get ready for the first case. This last patient is due to have a laparoscopic cholecystectomy. Rank the following options in order of appropriateness.

A. Explain to the registrar that this makes you feel uncomfortable.

B. Consent the patient.

C. Ask the registrar if you can watch him consent the patient to better understand the process.

D. Explain to the registrar that as an FY2 you will be unable to consent the patient.

E. Report the registrar to the GMC.

7. You are an FY2 doctor working in general practice. You see a patient with a suspected chest infection and prescribe them a course of antibiotics. After the patient leaves the room you realise that the patient's notes highlight a previous adverse reaction to the antibiotic you have prescribed. Rank the following in order of appropriateness.

A. Fill out a clinical incident form.

B. Reissue the patient with a different, more appropriate, antibiotic.

C. Highlight the case with your clinical supervisor.

D. Call the patient immediately to explain your mistake.

E. Wait until the end of clinic to call the patient so as not to delay your other patients' appointments.

8. You are asked to complete an online multi-source feedback form for your registrar. While you have no concerns about her clinical decision making, you do have some issues with her overall performance. Your registrar often turns up late to work and frequently uses humiliation as a teaching technique, which you have found upsetting. Rank the following in order of appropriateness.

A. Complete the feedback and use it as an opportunity to get back at your registrar by writing derogatory comments in her feedback.

B. Refuse to complete the form.

C. Complete the feedback and mention your concerns in a constructive way.

D. Make a reflective entry in your e-portfolio about the issues you have faced while working with this registrar.

E. Complete the rest of the form but only briefly comment on the issues of concern.

9. You are the FY2 on call for general medicine. At the time of handover you still have several jobs left on your list to do. On your way to your handover to the night team you are bleeped by one of the cardiology sisters who is concerned about a patient who has developed crushing central chest pain and has gone grey and clammy. Choose the **two** most appropriate options.

A. Attend the patient immediately and ask the sister to perform an ECG while you are on your way.

B. Go to handover and highlight the patient as an urgent case.

C. Ask the sister to call back in an hour to speak to the night FY2.

D. Attend the patient immediately.

E. Go to handover and routinely mention the patient to the night team.

10. You are an FY2 GP when a 25-year-old female patient presents requesting a termination of pregnancy. She and her partner had unprotected sexual intercourse six weeks ago and she has a positive pregnancy test. Your personal views mean that you have an objection to termination of pregnancy. Choose the **two** most appropriate options.

A. Refuse to see the patient ever again following this consultation

B. Express your disapproval of the patient's decision to terminate the pregnancy

C. Ask your supervisor for advice

D. Ensure that your personal views do not negatively impact on the patient's care

E. Sign the necessary documents even though it goes against your personal views

11. You are on a long haul flight when an announcement is made over the public address system asking for medical assistance because a fellow passenger has become unwell. A few minutes later, after no one has responded, you see the crew struggling to manage the medical emergency which is taking place on board. Which **three** of the following should you do?

A. Make yourself known to the crew and offer your assistance.

B. Attempt to save the patient's life at all costs, even if this means attempting a procedure you have no experience of.

C. Attempt to contact your defence union to check on your indemnity status before helping.

D. Comprehensively assess the patient to the best of your ability and training.

E. Discuss the case with the crew to decide on the most appropriate on-going management plan.

F. Do not make yourself known, but keep a watchful eye from afar to ensure that all is well.

12. You are working on a busy medical ward. In the rush of ordering an urgent CT scan for Mr Jones you accidently order it for Mr Smith, who is in the bed next to him. Unfortunately, by the time you notice your error Mr Smith has had the scan. Thankfully however, the scan is normal and shows no pathology. Rank the following in order of appropriateness.

A. Order a CT scan for Mr Jones.

B. Do not tell Mr Smith that an error has occurred as the scan was normal.

C. Speak to Mr Smith and apologise for the error.

D. Fill out an incident form.

E. Inform your supervising consultant.

13. While working as an A&E FY2 you see an 18-year-old patient who has presented with chest pain. He attends with his mother who is extremely anxious. You take a full history and explain the need for further tests. His mother leaves the cubicle to take a phone call and while she is away he tells you that he frequently takes cocaine. He asks you not to let his mother know. Having finished your history you leave the cubicle to order some more tests. At this point his mother finds you to ask if he admitted to taking drugs while she was gone as she has longstanding suspicions that he may be secretly taking drugs behind her back. Choose the **two** most appropriate actions.

A. Explain to her that there are many causes for chest pain.

B. Explain to her that her son has been taking cocaine.

C. Explain that you cannot discuss her son's case with her without him present as you would be in breach of confidentiality.

D. Explain that he has asked you not to tell his mother anything about what was said while she was gone.

E. Immediately call the police to report his drug usage.

F. Refuse to treat the patient further as his chest pain is likely self-inflicted.

G. Explain to his mother that her suspicions are correct but do not disclose which drug or how often he has taken it.

14. You are a GP FY2 doctor. A patient you have been seeing regularly has contacted you via a social media website. The private message asks if you would like to go for a social drink with them. Which **two** of the following would be most appropriate?

A. Write back to the patient and ask them not to contact you like this.

B. Write back to the patient and agree to go for a drink with them.

C. Talk to your supervisor about the issue.

D. Phone the patient at home and reprimand them for their actions.

E. Consult the GMC guidance on social media.

F. Ignore the message.

15. You are working as a GP FY2 doctor. You are running 30 minutes late for your appointments due to several complicated consultations. This is the third time this week that you have struggled to keep to time. When your next patient comes into your room they are extremely angry about the wait. They shout and scream about the delay and state that they are going to make a formal complaint. Rank the following in order of appropriateness.

A. Tell the patient that you will refuse to treat them unless they calm down.
B. Apologise to the patient for the delay.
C. Ask your supervising GP to come into the room to help defuse the situation.
D. Direct the patient to the practice complaints process.
E. Reflect with your trainer on ways to avoid running late during surgery.

16. You are helping your surgical registrar in theatre. She is new to the department and is doing her first unsupervised list of operations at this hospital. During the morning she becomes increasingly irritated by the scrub nurse who is unused to the way in which the registrar operates. On more than one occasion the registrar verbally criticises the nurse in front of the other theatre staff. At the end of the list the registrar storms off to the coffee room. The scrub nurse approaches you and asks you to speak with the registrar about her unacceptable behaviour. Rank the following in order of appropriateness.

A. Tell the nurse that it isn't your place to do this and she should speak to her senior.
B. Tell the nurse that you will speak to the registrar, but then deliberately avoid doing so.
C. Speak to the registrar and politely mention that the nurses were upset by what happened in theatre.
D. Speak to your consultant about the problem.
E. Report the registrar to the GMC for professional misconduct.

17. You are an FY2 and you are coming towards your end of year e-portfolio assessment. Due to some disorganisation on your part you have failed to get the correct number of "directly observed procedures" (DOPs) signed off in your portfolio. With your final sign-off looming rank the following in order of appropriateness.

A. Reflect on the reasons why you haven't made time to do these assessments earlier and make a reflective entry in your portfolio.
B. Arrange a time with your consultant to complete the required assessments.

C. Make no effort to get the assessments completed before your final sign off.

D. Log in and forge the assessments to make it look as though they have been completed in time.

E. Ask one of the medical registrars from another specialty if they could make time to directly observe you and complete the assessment accordingly.

18. You are an FY2 doctor and one of your fellow FY2s has been posting inappropriate public messages on a social media website. These messages initially were long rants about other colleagues from a variety of professions, but more recently she has posted some patient-identifiable information online. Rank the following actions in order of appropriateness.

A. Speak to the head of your foundation school about the issue.
B. Do nothing.
C. Talk to your colleague directly and advise her to delete the posts.
D. Direct your colleague to the GMC's guidance on doctors' use of social media.
E. Report your colleague to the GMC directly.

19. You are working in general practice when a patient you have been seeing for several months attends. He is thrilled with the quick diagnosis and referral you made for his skin cancer and as a token of his gratitude he has bought you a box of chocolates as a gift. Which **two** of the following actions would be the most appropriate?

A. Do not accept the gift and abruptly tell the patient not to do this again.
B. Seek advice from your supervisor about the practice's policy on receiving gifts from patients.
C. Ask the patient to make a donation to the practice instead.
D. Encourage the patient to bring more gifts in the future.
E. Accept the gift.
F. Accept the gift and ensure that the patient receives preferential treatment as a result.

20. A 23-year-old patient of yours has refused to inform the DVLA that he had an unprovoked epileptic seizure last month. Guidelines state that he must inform the DVLA and should not drive for a minimum of 6 months. You have seen him driving around town several times since you advised him not to. You are concerned that he may have another seizure whilst driving. Rank the following actions in order of appropriateness.

A. Break confidentiality and inform the DVLA directly yourself.
B. Reiterate to the patient that it is his responsibility to inform the DVLA.
C. Write to the patient to inform him that you will disclose their condition to the DVLA on their behalf if they continue to drive.
D. Under no circumstance break confidentiality.
E. Suggest that the patient asks for a second opinion.

21. You are a GP FY2 doctor. Seemingly unprovoked, a patient posts a derogatory review about your care on a well-known public website which many of your patients access. You are understandably upset by this, particularly as many of the facts regarding the case have been misrepresented in the review. Choose the **two** most appropriate options.

A. Discuss the situation with your clinical supervisor.
B. Discuss the situation with your medical defence union.
C. Respond in full on the website outlining the specific details of the case.
D. Ignore the comments.
E. Ask the practice manager to get the patient removed from the practice list to avoid any further incidents like this.

22. You are working as a GP FY2 doctor when a 22-year-old female patient presents. She is tearful and clearly distressed. She alleges that one of the senior partners at the practice (who is not your clinical supervisor) made several sexually inappropriate comments towards her during a consultation yesterday. Rank the following actions in order of appropriateness.

A. Discuss the case with your clinical supervisor immediately.
B. Seek advice from your medical defence union.
C. Call the police immediately.
D. Call the GMC to report the doctor.
E. Reassure the patient but take the allegations no further.

23. While out shopping at a supermarket, a patient you saw last week approaches you and tries to engage you in a discussion about their treatment and ongoing management plan. Several people are standing close by and can overhear your conversation. Choose the **two** most appropriate answers.

A. Politely explain to the patient that this is not the place to discuss their case.
B. Advise that should she wish to discuss her treatment further she should make an appointment to see you.
C. Take the patient to a quiet corner of the supermarket and answer her questions.

D. Ignore the patient.

E. Discuss the case but avoid mentioning any details.

24. While working in the rheumatology department as an FY2 doctor you are asked by your consultant to take a range of blood tests from an outpatient who will be reviewed again in clinic in 2 weeks' time with her results. You are unfamiliar with many of the blood tests that have been asked for. You dutifully take the blood tests and send the patient home. Later that day the laboratory phone you to inform you that one of the blood tests you have requested was sent to the lab in the wrong blood bottle and cannot be analysed. They advise you to take another sample. Rank the following in order of appropriateness.

A. Call the patient at home and inform them of what has happened.

B. Retake the sample when the patient attends for her follow up appointment.

C. Wait to see if the consultant notices there is no result for this investigation.

D. Arrange for a poster to be put up in the phlebotomy room outlining which tests belong in which blood bottles in order to avoid this error again.

E. Inform your consultant of your error.

25. You are an FY2 doctor on a busy surgical ward. Several tasks present themselves at once. Rank the tasks in the order that you would respond to them.

A. A patient has just returned from theatre and is found to be hypotensive and tachycardic. Their surgical drain is full of blood.

B. A patient in a side room is unresponsive and the nurse calls out as she cannot find a pulse.

C. A relative of one of your patients would like to speak to you because they feel that you have not told them enough about the management plan, despite the fact that you had a long conversation with them yesterday.

D. The biochemistry lab ask you to call them about one of your patients.

E. The ward clerk is very angry that you haven't done Mr Smith's discharge summary and hospital transport are here to collect him.

26. You are a GP FY2 doctor. At the end of a busy clinic you have five tasks remaining. Rank them in the order in which you would complete them.

   A. You need to dictate your routine referral letters from your morning clinic.

   B. You need to call your partner who has sent you a text message asking you to call them urgently.

   C. The receptionist tells you that there is a patient in the waiting room who is pale and complaining of chest pain.

   D. You need to start work on an audit which you have been putting off for weeks.

   E. You need to complete a telephone consultation with a patient with diabetes who has been unwell for twenty four hours and has now started vomiting.

27. You are working in a busy A&E department when one of your best friends from school presents with a minor ailment. He spots you in the waiting room and asks you if you will quickly see him so that he can skip the 4 hour long queue to be seen. Which **three** of the following are the most appropriate?

   A. Escort him discreetly into the A&E department and assess him yourself.

   B. Explain politely that you cannot do that.

   C. Tell him to go home and that you will visit him after your shift and assess him then.

   D. When his turn comes to be seen ask a colleague to see him instead of you.

   E. Abruptly explain his behaviour is inappropriate.

   F. Escort him discreetly into the A&E department and ask a colleague to see him.

   G. Maintain confidentiality about his attendance next time you see him socially.

28. You are about to start a job as the new psychiatry FY2 doctor. You have not done any clinical psychiatry since your placement in medical school and you are feeling very uncomfortable regarding your level of knowledge. In particular you are worried about the acute management of psychiatric conditions. Unfortunately, you are scheduled to be on call on your first day. Rank the following in the order in which you would do them.

   A. Phone the current psychiatry FY2 and ask them for advice on what common presentations you are likely to see when on call.

   B. Take time to read up on common acute psychiatric presentations.

   C. Assume that you will pick up the knowledge that you need as you go along.

    D. Explain your concerns to your supervising consultant and ask them about any resources that they would recommend.

    E. Make a "Personal Development Plan (PDP)" in your e-portfolio for your psychiatry placement.

29. You are a urology FY2. Your consultant is keen for you to gain experience in performing prostate examinations. He has suggested that you attend his theatre list in order to perform the examinations while the patients are under general anaesthetic so that it is less traumatic for the patients. Choose the **two** most appropriate statements, regarding patient consent, in this circumstance.

    A. Gain verbal consent from the patients to perform a rectal exam while they are under anaesthetic.

    B. Gain written consent from the patients to perform a rectal exam while they are under anaesthetic.

    C. Examine the patients under anaesthetic without consent.

    D. There is no need for further consent as the patient has consented to surgery.

    E. Consent can be acquired retrospectively.

30. You are the oncology FY2. A patient of yours, who happens to be a local celebrity, has sadly died from lymphoma despite several cycles of chemotherapy. The local paper is intending to print a front page tribute to the patient in tomorrow's issue. A reporter from the paper phones the ward and asks to speak to you. He wants to check his facts before the article goes to print and asks what type of lymphoma the patient had and whether it was the disease or a complication of treatment that caused the patient's death. Choose the **two** most appropriate actions.

    A. Explain that the death was not as a result of complications secondary to treatment.

    B. Answer any questions the reporter may have.

    C. Inform the reporter you are unable to give him any details at all.

    D. Inform your consultant of the reporter's call.

    E. Tell the reporter that it was Hodgkin lymphoma but that you cannot say anything else.

31. While working as a GP FY2, a patient presents to see you asking for a referral for a prophylactic bilateral mastectomy. She has no personal or family history of breast disease, and is not at increased risk of developing breast cancer. The patient explains that a well-known celebrity has recently had this treatment and she would also like to have it. You do not think that this treatment is appropriate. Rank the following in order of appropriateness.

A. Tell the patient that her request is inappropriate and refuse to discuss it further.
B. Refer the patient to a breast surgeon.
C. Explain to the patient that she has the right to ask for a second opinion.
D. Explore the patient's ideas, concerns and expectations further.
E. Ask your supervising GP for assistance.

32. You are an FY2 doctor. During your annual leave you visit your grandmother at home who is very unwell. She has metastatic bowel cancer and has been told by the palliative care consultant that she is in the final weeks of life. She has decided that she wants to die in her own home. When you see her she complains that her pain is becoming less well-controlled. Choose the **two** most appropriate answers.

A. Call her GP and inform him of the situation.
B. Call the medical registrar at the local hospital and arrange for admission.
C. Call an ambulance.
D. Prescribe regular oral analgesia.
E. Call the palliative care nurse and inform her of the situation.
F. Prescribe a syringe driver.

33. You are an A&E FY2. A 55-year-old farmer presents with a shotgun wound. He explains that his shotgun, which is fully licensed to him, accidentally discharged and shot him in the foot. Rank the following in order of appropriateness.

A. Call the police and inform them that there is a patient with a gunshot wound.
B. Treat the patient clinically.
C. Take advice from the duty consultant.
D. Call the police and give them the patient's details.
E. Do not call the police as the gun is licensed to the patient.

34. You are a GP FY2. You are called to do a home visit for a patient who has recently had a stroke. The patient, Mr Jones, is 55-years-old and was a professional sportsman in his youth. His stroke has left him wheelchair bound and requiring constant care. Understandably he has struggled to come to terms with his condition. During the consultation he becomes

tearful and asks you to kill him to stop his suffering. Rank the following in order of appropriateness.

A. Find out if Mr Jones has any symptoms that you could alleviate.
B. Suggest to Mr Jones that there are companies in mainland Europe who offer assisted dying.
C. Explore whether Mr Jones would like to discuss his feelings with a trained counsellor.
D. Explore Mr Jones' reasons for wanting to die.
E. Explain to Mr Jones that it would be illegal for you to kill him.

35. You are an A&E FY2. One of the staff nurses asks to speak to you privately. She explains that she has experienced some weight loss and has had some small amounts of blood in her stools over the last few months. Her father died of bowel cancer and she is worried. She asks if you might be able to examine her and order the tests needed to investigate her problem. Choose the **two** most appropriate actions.

A. Advise the nurse to see her GP about the problem.
B. Advise the nurse to book herself into A&E as a patient.
C. Scold the nurse for her unprofessional behaviour.
D. Arrange an urgent CT scan of her abdomen and pelvis.
E. Advise the nurse that it is probably a benign problem and not to worry.
F. Advise the nurse that you cannot examine her as it would be inappropriate.

36. You are a surgical FY2. A 35-year-old patient on the ward underwent a large surgical procedure yesterday and has suffered from significant post-operative bleeding today. She is due to return to theatre today to stem the bleeding. The consultant surgeon would like her to have a blood transfusion during the operation. The patient does not want this to happen on religious grounds as she is a Jehovah's Witness. Choose the **two** most appropriate answers.

A. Transfuse the patient with blood while she is under general anaesthetic.
B. Ensure the patient is fully informed of the implications of her decision.
C. Explore alternative treatment options which might be able to avoid transfusion.
D. Refuse to treat the patient.
E. Treat the patient against her wishes, in her "best interest".

37. You are an A&E FY2. You attend an elderly patient who is very unwell and dies suddenly in the A&E department. You are very upset by this and discuss the case with the consultant in the department who assures you that you did everything you could have done. Despite this your confidence is affected substantially. You begin to feel nervous about seeing acutely unwell patients on your own and dread going to work. Recently you have had recurring nightmares about the case. Choose the **two** most appropriate options.

    A. Speak to your clinical supervisor about the issues you are having.
    B. Try to avoid seeing very sick patients on your own for a while.
    C. Try to forget about the case by socialising and drinking more outside of work.
    D. Approach your deanery's counselling service.
    E. Try to carry on working despite how you are feeling.

38. You are a GP FY2. A patient who is new to the practice attends and demands that you prescribe him oral morphine. He gives no reason for this and becomes verbally abusive when you do not immediately sign a prescription. Rank the following in order of appropriateness.

    A. Prescribe the oral morphine immediately.
    B. Ask your supervisor for help in managing the situation.
    C. Remain calm and polite.
    D. Try to explore why the patient has made the request.
    E. Tell the patient that you will refuse to treat him if he continues to be abusive.

39. You are an FY2 when one of the nurses approaches you to discuss the FY1 doctor on your team. The nurses find him to be very rude and abrasive and earlier today he upset one of the healthcare assistants. The nurse wants you to do something about it. Choose the **three** most appropriate options.

    A. Have a quiet word with the FY1 to discuss the issues raised.
    B. Explain to the nurse that she should speak to the doctor herself.
    C. Ask your registrar for advice on how to deal with the situation.
    D. Tell the FY1 that his behaviour is unacceptable while on the ward so that the nurses can hear your conversation.
    E. Reassure the nurse that you will take her concerns seriously.
    F. Report the FY1 to the foundation school.
    G. Do nothing.

40. You are driving home from work when a car in front of you hits a cyclist at speed. Clearly the cyclist is severely injured. Rank the following in order of importance.

    A. Treat the cyclist to the best of your ability.
    B. Pull over to help, but ensure that you are safe when doing so.
    C. Contact your defence union to ask them about your medico–legal cover for acting in such a situation.
    D. Ask another bystander to call an ambulance.
    E. Do nothing.

41. While walking across the hospital car park one evening after work you find a patient list on the floor. Although the date on the list is from a month ago it has all the medical details of the patients who were on one of the surgical wards. Clearly this has been accidentally dropped by another member of the medical team. Choose the **two** most appropriate actions.

    A. Inform the hospital's clinical governance lead.
    B. Leave the list where it is.
    C. Pick the list up and dispose of it when you get home.
    D. After disposing of the list take the matter no further.
    E. Take the list back into the hospital and put it in a confidential waste bin.

42. You are working as a GP FY2. While you are on a home visit you leave your doctor's bag, which contains some drugs, and the patient's notes in your car. To your horror, when you return you find that your car has been stolen. Rank the following in order of appropriateness.

    A. Call the police.
    B. Arrange for a replacement vehicle.
    C. Inform the patient as to what has happened.
    D. Inform your supervisor.
    E. Complete an incident form.

43. You have just started your post as a respiratory FY2. You have not had to interpret any arterial blood gas (ABG) results for several months as your previous post was as part of the psychiatry team. As a consequence you feel very unconfident in interpreting ABGs on your own. Rank the following actions in order of appropriateness.

    A. Try to do some further reading about ABG interpretation.
    B. Do nothing.

C. Speak to your registrar about your concerns.

D. Undertake an e-learning module in ABG interpretation.

E. Try to improve your knowledge of ABGs by picking up tips over the coming months.

44. While working on a general medical ward you start to notice that the nurse practitioner in your team is increasingly critical of your work. Initially her comments pertained to your clinical decision making, but recently her remarks have become more personal. Understandably this has begun to upset you and affect your confidence. Choose the **two** most appropriate actions.

   A. Report the nurse practitioner to the Nursing and Midwifery Council.

   B. Speak to your clinical supervisor about the issue.

   C. Do nothing.

   D. Speak to the nurse practitioner directly about the problem.

   E. Report the nurse practitioner to the head of nursing.

45. While working on a general surgical ward a patient of yours is diagnosed with inoperable pancreatic cancer and is told that he likely has only weeks to live. At the multidisciplinary team meeting the patient's case is discussed and it is concluded that palliative chemotherapy may extend the prognosis to a maximum of 6 months. However, the patient decides that he does not want any chemotherapy due to the potential side effects and would rather let the disease take its natural course. Rank the following in order of appropriateness.

   A. Inform the patient's GP of his decision.

   B. Explore the patient's understanding of the situation.

   C. Respect the patient's decision.

   D. Give the patient chemotherapy as it is "in his best interests".

   E. Answer any questions the patient may have.

46. You are a GP FY2. A 54-year-old man presents to clinic complaining of stress. Earlier this week you saw his wife, who is also one of your patients. She said that her husband had assaulted her last week during an argument. You suspect that the patient may be subjecting his wife to domestic violence. Rank the following in order of appropriateness.

   A. Explain to the patient that his wife mentioned that he assaulted her last week.

   B. Discuss how his stress is affecting his life.

   C. Discuss the case with your clinical supervisor.

D. Find out if there are any children at home.

E. Explore the patient's reasons for being stressed.

47. You are an FY2 on a morning surgical ward round with a locum registrar who you have not met before. Several times during the round he leaves the curtains open during consultations and you haven't seen him wash his hands once between patients. Rank the following in order of appropriateness.

A. Pull the curtains around the cubicles yourself.

B. Continue with the ward round and do not raise these issues.

C. Speak to your consultant about these issues.

D. Report the registrar to the GMC.

E. Mention to the registrar that he should wash his hands.

48. You are an FY2 doctor working on a busy surgical ward. You have a long list of jobs to complete following the morning ward round and you are feeling stressed. At the end of the round your consultant asks you to mentor a final year medical student for the day. Choose the **two** most appropriate options.

A. Refuse to mentor the student and explain that you are too busy.

B. Agree to mentor the student.

C. Ask the student to complete some of the jobs you have to do.

D. Ask the student to complete the jobs that you don't want to do.

E. Find out what learning objectives the student has and try to meet them.

49. You are an FY2 working in cardiology. You have been asked by your consultant to prescribe an infusion of a drug that you are unfamiliar with and have never prescribed before. Rank the following in order of appropriateness.

A. Consult the BNF for guidance on how to prescribe the drug.

B. Attempt to prescribe the drug as best you can without further help.

C. Consult the hospital's protocol for the drug.

D. Ask your registrar for help in prescribing the drug.

E. Do not prescribe the drug.

50. You are one of two urology FY2s working together in the same team. Your colleague hands over to you from the night shift and goes home. A short while later you receive a phone call asking you to review a patient with a urological emergency who was admitted overnight. The A&E doctor explains that your colleague who was on call overnight said that she would hand the patient over to the day team for review. However, you received no such

handover and know nothing about the patient. Rank the following in order of appropriateness.

A. Speak to your colleague about why she did not hand the patient over.
B. Go to see the patient straight away.
C. Refuse to see the patient as they were not handed over from the night team.
D. Speak to your consultant about the issue.
E. Complete an incident form.

51. While walking down one of the corridors in your hospital a man in front of you collapses suddenly. After initially assessing the patient you conclude that the patient is in cardiac arrest. You are the only doctor nearby, and there are several passers-by who have stopped to look at the commotion. Which of the following would be the first **two** things you would do?

A. Berate the bystanders for watching the emergency unfold.
B. Begin cardiopulmonary resuscitation (CPR).
C. Discuss the case with your clinical supervisor.
D. Ask one of the bystanders to call "2222" and request the "crash team".
E. Order an urgent CT scan to rule out a pulmonary embolus.
F. Transfer the man to the cardiac catheter laboratory.

52. You are the FY2 on a busy general medical ward. The ward clerk asks to speak to you as she is deeply unhappy at how slowly you complete your discharge summaries. She shows you a pile of ten outstanding discharge summaries for patients who went home last week. Rank the following in order of appropriateness.

A. Explain to the ward clerk that you have much more pressing tasks to attend to than completing discharge summaries.
B. Apologize to the ward clerk and explain that you will resolve the backlog of discharges as soon as you can.
C. Reflect on why so many discharge summaries have gone unwritten in order to improve your efficiency.
D. Ask some of the other members of your team to help you complete the outstanding discharge summaries.
E. Complete the outstanding discharge summaries as quickly as possible even if that means that they are inaccurate.

53. You are an FY2 on a placement in primary care when a patient attends to request a note to explain to his employer that he is sick. Undoubtedly the patient has tonsillitis but he is likely to be unwell for only a few days. The patient is unperturbed by this advice and demands that you write him a "sick note." Choose the **two** most appropriate options.

A. Give the patient advice on supportive measures to aid his symptoms.
B. Give the patient a note for 2 weeks.
C. Give the patient a note for 1 week.
D. Explain to the patient that he can self–certificate for up to 7 days.
E. Give the patient a blank note so that he can enter the date that he goes back to work himself.

54. You are an FY2 in primary care. You are called to a home visit for an elderly patient who has requested a home visit that morning as she has been feeling unwell for the last 24 hours. She has not been seen by any of the doctors at the surgery for several months. When you attend the patient's house there is no answer but the door is unlocked. You enter only to find that the patient has died in bed. Rank the following actions in the order you should do them.

A. Contact the coroner.
B. Call your supervisor for advice.
C. Contact the police.
D. Confirm that there are no signs of life.
E. Inform the next of kin.

55. A patient presents to you in a general medical clinic. They have some excellent clinical signs which you think would be useful to help teach medical students in the future. Therefore you are keen to take some pictures of the patient for educational purposes. Rank the following in order of appropriateness.

A. Explain to the patient why you would like to take the photographs.
B. Gain written consent to take the images.
C. Contact the medical photography department to arrange the photographs.
D. Take the pictures on your phone and upload them to your computer.
E. Gain oral consent to take the images.

| Clinical Problem Solving paper

100 Questions

Time Limit: 75 minutes

1. A 35-year-old man presents with an acutely painful red left eye. He has some blurred vision and photophobia. Examination reveals a hypopyon in the left anterior chamber. He has a past medical history of ankylosing spondylitis. Choose the most likely diagnosis.

   A. Dendritic ulcer
   B. Anterior uveitis
   C. Allergic conjunctivitis
   D. Acute closed angle glaucoma
   E. Scleritis

2. A 50-year-old female patient has developed lethargy and weight gain associated with excessive milky discharge from her breasts. She has also recently developed headaches. As part of her assessment you examine her visual fields. What is the most likely clinical finding?

   A. Homonymous hemianopia
   B. Quadrantanopia
   C. Central scotoma
   D. Bitemporal haemianopia
   E. Unilateral visual loss

3. A 27-year-old pregnant mother presents as she is about to travel abroad to visit family. She would like to know which vaccinations she can safely receive whilst pregnant. Which one of the following vaccines can the patient safely receive during her pregnancy?

   A. Rubella
   B. Pertussis
   C. Mumps
   D. Measles
   E. BCG

4. A 39-year-old female patient presents with a three month history of post-coital bleeding. She has never attended a routine smear appointment and is

worried this might represent cervical cancer. Which of the following is **not** a recognised risk factor for cervical cancer?

A. Human parainfluenza virus

B. Smoking

C. Early age of first sexual intercourse

D. Multiple sexual partners

E. Immunosuppression

5. You are an FY2 in A&E when a 45-year-old patient becomes acutely unwell after being administered an intravenous drug. He becomes short of breath with marked wheeze and cardiovascular collapse. He develops a widespread rash and facial swelling. You suspect anaphylaxis. What is the most appropriate initial management?

A. 500 mcg of 1:1000 adrenaline I.M.

B. 1mg of 1:10,000 adrenaline I.M.

C. 500mcg of 1:1000 adrenaline I.V.

D. 1mg of 1:10,000 adrenaline I.V.

E. 1mg of 1:1000 adrenaline I.V.

6. A 23-year-old male patient presents with an acute asthma attack. Which of the following features would suggest that his asthma attack is life-threatening?

A. Respiratory rate >25/min

B. PEF 33–50% of best or predicted

C. Heart rate >110 bpm

D. Inability to complete sentences in one breath

E. Altered conscious level

7. A 65-year-old male patient attends for a routine appointment. He is found to be hypertensive. After serial blood pressure measurements over a number of weeks you diagnose him with essential hypertension. Assuming no contraindications, what would be the most appropriate first line pharmacological management for this patient?

A. Doxazocin

B. Amlodipine

C. Bisoprolol

D. Bendroflumethiazide

E. Ramipril

8, 9, 10. Regarding drugs used in cardiology:

    A. Aspirin
    B. Warfarin
    C. Propranolol
    D. Furosemide
    E. Amlodipine
    F. Clopidogrel
    G. Ramipril
    H. Bendroflumethiazide

For each of the following scenarios choose the drug from the above list which would be most likely to cause the side-effect described. Each option can be used once, more than once, or not at all.

8. A 75-year-old man presents with swelling of the face, lips and tongue, within a few weeks of starting a new medication.

9. An 80-year-old patient is commenced on a new medication and notices increased swelling of her ankles and feet.

10. A 65-year-old female patient is concerned that since starting her new medication she has experienced cold fingers and toes made worse when she goes outside.

11. A 60-year-old female presents acutely with worsening pain and weakness in her muscles. Blood tests revealed a markedly raised creatine kinase. The patient is currently taking several medications. Which of the following drug interactions is most likely to explain the patient's presentation?

    A. Simvastatin and Amlodipine
    B. Simvastatin and Aspirin
    C. Amlodipine and Aspirin
    D. Clarithromycin and Simvastatin
    E. Clarithromycin and Amlodipine

12, 13, 14. Regarding abdominal pain:

    A. Ascending Cholangitis
    B. Pancreatic Cancer
    C. Cholecystitis
    D. Biliary Colic
    E. Gallstone Ileus
    F. Cholelithiasis
    G. Pancreatitis
    H. Renal Colic

For each of the following scenarios choose the option from the above list which would be the most likely diagnosis or symptom. Each option can be used once, more than once, or not at all.

12. A 45-year-old patient develops severe epigastric pain one day after undergoing endoscopic retrograde cholangiopancreatography (ERCP). Her amylase level is markedly raised.

13. A 60-year-old overweight female patient develops severe spasmodic pain which is maximal in the right upper quadrant. She has had this pain before and associates it with eating fatty meals. She is otherwise systemically well and her blood tests are normal.

14. A 58-year-old male is undergoing a routine abdominal ultrasound. He is clinically well and the scan finds no abnormality other than an incidental finding of asymptomatic gallstones within the gall bladder.

15. A 35-year-old female patient presents with a 3 month history of lethargy. She feels tired all the time and it is starting to have an effect on her ability to work. You note that she appears very pale with pale conjunctivae. She mentions that for more than a year she has been bleeding excessively when menstruating. Which of the following would be the most likely finding when examining her nails?

A. Koilonychia
B. Onycholysis
C. Nail pitting
D. Clubbing
E. Splinter haemorrhages

16. A 6-year-old boy with asthma presents with dry itchy skin affecting the flexor surfaces of his arms and legs. You diagnose him with atopic eczema. Which of the following would be the most appropriate first line treatment?

A. Phototherapy
B. Topical calcineurin inhibitors
C. Potent topical steroids
D. Emollients
E. Systemic therapy

17. A 57-year-old patient presents with dizziness. She describes frequent episodes, lasting for a few seconds when rolling over in bed or turning her head suddenly. These episodes are often associated with nausea and the sensation that the room is rotating. What is the most likely diagnosis?

A. Acoustic Neuroma
B. Vestibular Neuronitis
C. Ménière's Syndrome
D. Transient Ischaemic Attack
E. Benign Paroxysmal Positional Vertigo (BPPV)

18. A 75-year-old male patient presents with sudden painless monocular visual loss in the left eye. The patient has a past medical history of diabetes and atrial fibrillation. Fundoscopy reveals a hypopigmented retina with a well-defined red dot at the area of the macula.

A. Central retinal vein occlusion
B. Amaurosis fugax
C. Retinal detachment
D. Central retinal artery occlusion
E. Retinal detachment

19. A 55-year-old man presents with lethargy, polydipsia and polyuria for several months. He is overweight and there is a strong family history of diabetes mellitus. You measure a random venous plasma glucose level which is raised (16 mmol/l). In order to formally diagnose this patient with diabetes mellitus what would be the next most appropriate step?

A. No further investigations required
B. A fasting plasma glucose measurement
C. Oral Glucose Tolerance test
D. HbA1c test
E. Repeat random venous plasma glucose level

20. A 20-year-old patient presents with fatigue, myalgia and weight loss. She has a past medical history of hypothyroidism and also has vitiligo. On examination the patient has increased pigmentation in the palmar creases and buccal mucosa. You suspect Addison's disease. Which of the following would you expect to find in this patient?

A. Hypernatraemia
B. Hypocalcaemia
C. Hyperkalaemia
D. Hyperglycaemia
E. Lymphopenia

21, 22, 23.   Regarding lumps in the scrotum:

   A.   Hydrocele
   B.   Indirect inguinal hernia
   C.   Varicocele
   D.   Testicular tumour
   E.   Haematoma
   F.   Testicular torsion
   G.   Spermatocele
   H.   Direct inguinal hernia

   For each of the following scenarios choose the option from the above list which would be the most likely diagnosis. Each option can be used once, more than once, or not at all.

21.   A 23-year-old male university student presents in an anxious state as he has noticed a lump in his scrotum during self-examination. On examination there is a smooth, well demarcated mass superior to the testicle. The mass transilluminates when a light source is placed behind it.

22.   A 19-year-old male patient presents with a right sided scrotal swelling which is causing a dragging sensation. The patient has also been experiencing some back pain recently. On examination there is a large mass in the right hemiscrotum which is hard and craggy. You cannot feel a normal testicle on that side, although the left testicle is normal.

23.   A 7-year-old boy presents with sudden onset severe testicular and abdominal pain with vomiting. On examination he has a high-riding right sided testicle which is red and he will not allow anyone to touch it.

24.   A 55-year-old patient presents acutely with severe epigastric pain radiating through to his back shortly after commencing a new diabetic medication. Which of the following medications is most likely to have caused these symptoms?

   A.   Pioglitazone
   B.   Gliclazide
   C.   Insulin
   D.   Metformin
   E.   Sitagliptin

25.   A 75-year-old patient presents with sudden onset shortness of breath. He is tachypnoeic and his ECG shows a sinus tachycardia of 110bpm. Oxygen saturations on room air are 90% and his JVP is raised. His only past medical history is prostate cancer which has unfortunately metastasised and for which he is now being treated palliatively. What is the most likely diagnosis?

A. Pneumonia
B. Congestive cardiac failure
C. Pulmonary embolus
D. Myocardial infarction
E. Pneumothorax

26. A 10-year-old boy, with no past medical history, presents with abdominal pain. He has been unwell with vague abdominal pain and vomiting for the last 24 hours. His mother tells you that he has had a temperature and is off his food. On examining the patient there is rebound tenderness and guarding over the right iliac fossa. What is the most likely diagnosis?

A. Intussusception
B. Mesenteric adenitis
C. Reflux oesophagitis
D. Gastroenteritis
E. Appendicitis

27, 28, 29. Regarding genetic syndromes:

A. Patau's syndrome
B. Prader-Willi syndrome
C. Di George syndrome
D. Edwards' syndrome
E. Turner's syndrome
F. Angelman syndrome
G. Down syndrome
H. Klinefelter's syndrome

For each of the following patient descriptions choose the option from the above list which would be the most likely diagnosis. Each option can be used once, more than once, or not at all.

27. A 3-month-old baby has low set ears and a small jaw. The child has a short and prominent sternum with widely spaced nipples. His fingers are clenched and noticeably overlap each other. His big toes are flexed and the heels of his feet are particularly prominent.

28. A 7-year-old girl is particularly short for her age. She has a noticeably broad chest and has marked webbing of the neck. She has a past medical history of aortic coarctation.

29. A 5-year-old boy has a flattened occiput and facial appearance. He has a single palmar crease and prominent epicanthal folds.

30, 31, 32. Regarding drug overdose

    A. Cyproheptadine
    B. Flumazenil
    C. N-acetylcysteine
    D. Glucagon
    E. Octreotide
    F. Naloxone
    G. Deferoxamine
    H. Protamine sulphate

For each of the following patients choose the option from the above list which would be the most appropriate treatment. Each option can be used once, more than once or not at all.

30. A 30-year-old patient presents to A&E after taking an overdose of codeine.

31. A 30-year-old patient presents to A&E after taking an overdose of diazepam.

32. A 30-year-old patient presents to A&E after taking an overdose of paracetamol.

33. A female patient presents with some unexpected uterine bleeding. She is concerned that this may represent endometrial cancer and wants a referral to see a gynaecologist. As part of your discussion you explore risk factors. Which of the following options has not been shown to increase the risk of developing endometrial cancer?

    A. Obesity
    B. Unopposed Oestrogen Therapy
    C. Combined oral contraceptive pill (COCP)
    D. Tamoxifen
    E. Polycystic Ovarian Syndrome

34. A 36-year-old primiparous female patient wants to start contraception. She is clinically well and her only past medical history is fibroids. She smokes 20 cigarettes per day. During your discussion about contraception, she confides in you that she is extremely needle-phobic. Which of the following would be the most appropriate contraception for this patient?

    A. Progesterone only pill (POP)
    B. Mirena intrauterine system
    C. Combined oral contraceptive pill (COCP)
    D. Implanon
    E. Depo–Provera

35. You are an FY2 doctor in general practice. An 18-year-old female patient with acne presents to you because she is concerned about the potential side effects of Isotretinoin (a retinoid drug), which was recently prescribed by her dermatologist. Which of the following is not a recognised side effect of this drug?

    A. Oily skin
    B. Teratogenicity
    C. Increased sensitivity to sunlight
    D. Anaemia
    E. Leucopenia

36. An 80-year-old Iranian man presents with a three month history of dysphagia. Initially the patient was struggling to swallow solid food, but over the last few weeks this has gradually progressed and he is now also having difficulty swallowing fluids. He has little past medical history of note but has smoked an average of 20 cigarettes every day since he was 15 years old and drinks 40 units of alcohol per week. He has lost 15kg in weight since symptoms began and blood tests show that he is anaemic. What is the most likely cause for his dysphagia?

    A. Chagas' disease
    B. Stroke
    C. Achalasia
    D. Thoracic aortic aneurysm
    E. Oesophageal cancer

37, 38, 39. Regarding the urinary tract:

    A. Orthostatic proteinuria
    B. Normal pregnancy
    C. Nephrotic syndrome
    D. Bladder cancer
    E. Nephritic syndrome
    F. Prostate cancer
    G. Pre-eclampsia
    H. Pregnancy induced hypertension

For each of the following scenarios choose the option from the above list which would be the most likely diagnosis. Each option can be used once, more than once, or not at all.

37. A 75-year-old man presents with painless macroscopic haematuria. He has little past medical history of note. He is a lifelong smoker and worked in the textiles industry for over forty years.

38. An 18-year-old primigravida patient presents to you at 32 weeks as she is feeling unwell with a headache. A urine dipstick shows proteinuria but is negative for blood or infection. Her blood pressure is 170/105. What is the most likely diagnosis?

39. A 16-year-old male patient was found to have proteinuria on a routine urine dipstick. Blood tests including renal function tests were all normal. Additionally, a renal ultrasound scan was normal. On further investigation the patient's morning urine samples are always negative for protein. However, samples taken later in the day are always positive.

40. An 80-year-old with sepsis secondary to severe pneumonia is brought into A&E by ambulance in a confused state. When you assess her Glasgow Coma Score (GCS) she obeys commands but will not open her eyes and continuously mutters inappropriate words. What is her GCS?

A. 9
B. 10
C. 11
D. 12
E. 13

41. You are working on a general medical ward when a patient is given a dose of penicillin. The patient becomes acutely unwell with bronchospasm and wheeze. She quickly develops facial oedema and a widespread rash. You suspect anaphylaxis. Which of the following would be compatible with this reaction?

A. Type I hypersensitivity
B. Type II hypersensitivity
C. Type III hypersensitivity
D. Type IV hypersensitivity
E. Type V hypersensitivity

42. A 75-year-old patient presents to you in general practice because she has a feeling of "something coming down" when she defecates. She explains that on more than one occasion she has needed to replace the mass herself. Apart from COPD and four normal vaginal deliveries, she has no other past medical history. On examination, she clearly has prolapsed haemorrhoids which are manually reducible and not thrombosed. However, they do not reduce spontaneously. What is the most appropriate description of this patient's problem?

    A. Normal
    B. 1st degree haemorrhoids
    C. 2nd degree haemorrhoids
    D. 3rd degree haemorrhoids
    E. 4th degree haemorrhoids

43. A 30-year-old man with an extensive psychiatric history presents for a routine appointment. In the past he has had several suicide attempts and frequently attends the local A&E with episodes of self-harm. He finds it difficult to control his emotions and often acts impulsively. He has been known to occasionally hear voices when undergoing periods of stress. These stressful periods often arise after the breakdown of one of his many intense but brief relationships. Which of the following diagnoses is the most likely in this case?

    A. Dependent personality disorder
    B. Narcissistic personality disorder
    C. Anakastic personality disorder
    D. Paranoid personality disorder
    E. Borderline personality disorder

44. A 50-year-old overweight man presents in agony with an acutely tender foot. On examination the first metatarsophalangeal joint is erythematous, warm to touch and excruciatingly tender. He is otherwise clinically well with no past medical history of note. You suspect he has developed gout. Assuming no contraindications, what would be the most appropriate acute management?

    A. Diclofenac
    B. Intra-articular steroid injection
    C. Allopurinol
    D. Intravenous morphine
    E. Oral steroids

45. An 80-year-old patient presents acutely because he is worried that he has had a stroke. He developed sudden onset slurring of his words which lasted for approximately 5 minutes. He had no other neurological deficit at that time and all of his symptoms have now fully resolved. He has no past medical history of note. On examination, he has a regular pulse of 72bpm and a blood pressure of 155/85. You suspect he has had a transient ischaemic attack (TIA). While trying to establish the most appropriate management you calculate his ABCD2 score. What is this patient's ABCD2 score?

A. Zero
B. One
C. Two
D. Three
E. Four

46, 47, 48. Regarding headache:

A. Tension type headache
B. Migraine
C. Cluster headache
D. Thunderclap
E. Coital cephalgia
F. Sinusitis
G. Withdrawal headache
H. Hemicrania continua

For each of the following scenarios chose the most appropriate option from the list above. Each option may be used once, more than once, or not at all.

46. A 35-year-old male presents because of a bout of recent headaches. The patient describes a severe unilateral headache which has, on occasion, woken him from sleep. The pain is often associated with eye-watering and a sensation of nasal blockage. Until these recent episodes, he hadn't had headaches like these for several months. He is a smoker but has no other past medical history.

47. A 40-year-old woman presents because of recent headaches. She describes a severe headache which is like a "tight band" around her head. She has no other associated symptoms at all and the pain seems to worsen as the day progresses, becoming maximal in the evening.

48. A 20-year-old university student presents with a unilateral throbbing headache which is associated with nausea and on one occasion an episode of vomiting. The patient says that on each occasion the headache is preceded by "zig-zags" in her vision.

49. During genetic counselling a prospective mother and father are both found to be carriers of the autosomal recessive cystic fibrosis gene. They want to know the likelihood of them having a child who suffers from cystic fibrosis. Choose the most appropriate answer.

   A. 0%
   B. 25%
   C. 50%
   D. 75%
   E. 100%

50. An anxious mother and father attend for advice regarding the impending birth of their first child. They have been told that they are expecting a boy. The father suffers from Haemophilia A (X-linked recessive). They would like to know what the likelihood is of their son inheriting the disease from him. Choose the most appropriate answer.

   A. 0%
   B. 25%
   C. 50%
   D. 75%
   E. 100%

51. A 45-year-old patient presents to you in primary care with low mood. Since losing his mother to cancer 4 months ago he has become increasingly despondent and unmotivated and this has now resulted in him losing his job. He is clearly tearful. He has decided to seek medical help and you suspect that he is suffering from depression. In order to gain an objective measure of his mood which one of the following patient questionnaires would be most helpful in this case?

   A. AUDIT
   B. PDI
   C. PHQ-9
   D. QCPC
   E. PSQ

52. An 80-year-old man is admitted to hospital in a confused state. His wife says his memory has been getting worse recently. You suspect that the patient

either has delirium or dementia. Which of the following features would be most consistent with a diagnosis of delirium?

A. Acute onset over hours or days
B. Progressive
C. Lasting for months/years
D. Normal attention
E. Irreversible

53. You are asked to see a 65-year-old man with advanced metastatic prostate cancer at his home. Over the last few days he has become increasingly weak. He has gone from being able to walk around the house to not being able to stand up. Neurological examination reveals that he has numbness over the buttocks, marked weakness in all movements in the lower legs and absent ankle reflexes. Additionally, he has reduced anal tone and appears to be in urinary retention. What is the most appropriate next step?

A. Review the patient in one week's time.
B. Review the patient again tomorrow.
C. Refer the patient routinely to the urology team.
D. Refer the patient urgently to the urology team.
E. Admit the patient acutely under the neurosurgical team.

54, 55, 56. Regarding the nerves of the arm and hand:

A. Radial nerve
B. Palmar digital nerves
C. Medial cutaneous nerve
D. Median nerve
E. Axillary nerve
F. Ulnar nerve
G. Musculocutaneous nerve
H. Subclavian nerve

For each of the following scenarios choose the option from the above list which would be the most likely nerve affected in each scenario. Each option can be used once, more than once, or not at all.

54. A 25-year-old pregnant patient with gestational diabetes presents with a history of discomfort and paraesthesia in the thumb, index, middle and lateral half of the ring finger of her right hand. She describes symptoms which are worse at night and improve when she shakes her hand vigorously. On examination she has some wasting of the thenar muscles of the affected hand and Tinel's test is positive.

55. An 80-year-old patient presents to A&E following a fall while out shopping. She has suffered a fracture to the midshaft of her right humerus. Examination of her arm reveals that she cannot extend her hand at the wrist (wrist drop).

56. A 20-year-old rugby player presents to A&E with an anterior dislocation of the left shoulder. Neurological examination of the arm before relocation of the joint shows a well demarcated area of numbness over the inferior deltoid.

57. An 80-year-old presents with a troublesome finger. She has noticed over recent weeks that the ring finger on her right hand frequently gets stuck in flexion. She describes how she uses her left hand to forcibly extend the finger. On examination there is a small, but palpable nodule on the palmar surface of the affected finger. What is the most likely diagnosis?

A. Mallet finger
B. Gamekeeper's thumb
C. De Quervain's tenosynovitis
D. Trigger finger
E. Dupuytren's contracture

58. A 50-year-old male presents to A&E with chest pain. He was seen in the department two weeks ago with a myocardial infarction, and was only discharged from the cardiology ward last week. He has been pyrexial and has developed chest pain. A bedside echocardiogram reveals a pericardial effusion. What is the most likely diagnosis?

A. Tietze syndrome
B. Dressler's syndrome
C. Hurler syndrome
D. Hunter syndrome
E. Dubin–Johnson syndrome

59, 60, 61. Regarding hernias:

A. Incisional hernia
B. Spigelian hernia
C. Indirect inguinal hernia
D. Parastomal hernia
E. Paraumbilical hernia
F. Obturator hernia
G. Femoral hernia
H. Direct inguinal hernia

For each of the following scenarios choose the option from the above list which would be the most likely diagnosis. Each option can be used once, more than once, or not at all.

59. A 20-year-old man presents with a right-sided mass in his groin. On examination the mass is easily reduced and pressure over the internal inguinal ring prevents it from reappearing.

60. A 55-year-old female patient presents with a painless abdominal mass which arises just superiorly to the umbilicus in the midline. It is irreducible but not painful.

61. A 55-year-old man with a past medical history of bowel cancer and obesity presents with a painless abdominal mass. He has noticed that in recent months a swelling has developed around the site of his colostomy. It is more noticeable when standing and resolves when he is lying flat.

62. A 30-year-old male patient presents with a slight yellowing of the sclera of his eyes. He first noticed this change two days ago while he was experiencing some cold-like symptoms. He is otherwise clinically well with no past medical history and drinks only 6 units of alcohol per week. He has a normal clinical examination. Blood test show normal liver function tests (LFTs) with the exception of a very mildly raised bilirubin. What is the most likely diagnosis?

    A. Acute liver failure
    B. Decompensated alcoholic liver disease
    C. Non-alcoholic steatohepatitis
    D. Gilbert's syndrome
    E. Autoimmune hepatitis

63. A 55-year-old patient presents because he has noticed a creamy yellow lesion in his left eye. On examination, the triangular lesion is raised and well demarcated on the nasal side of the sclera of the left eye. It does not encroach onto the cornea. The patient has recently returned from several years living in Australia. What is the most likely diagnosis?

    A. Pinguecula
    B. Corneal abrasion
    C. Iritis
    D. Scleritis
    E. Pterygium

64. A 21-year-old female patient presents with acute tonsillitis. She is demanding antibiotics because she needs to get back to work as soon as possible. In order to assess the appropriateness of prescribing her antibiotics you use the Centor criteria to guide you on the likelihood of this being a streptococcal tonsillitis. Which one of the following is not part of the Centor criteria?

A. Presence of tonsillar exudate
B. Presence of cervical lymphadenopathy
C. Presence of fever (>38 degrees Celsius)
D. Presence of immunosuppression
E. Absence of cough

65. You are working in general practice when you are called out on a domiciliary visit to see a 15-year-old boy who has been unwell with headache, vomiting and photophobia. When you arrive at the patient's house he has marked meningism and an evolving petechial rash. You have a strong suspicion of meningococcal meningitis. After calling for an ambulance, and assuming no allergy, which of the following would be the most appropriate drug to administer?

A. I.M. Benzylpenicillin
B. P.O. Flucloxacillin
C. I.M. Gentamicin
D. I.V. Clarithromycin
E. I.M. Chloramphenicol

66. You are working in A&E when a patient who has been in a road traffic collision presents via ambulance. During your initial assessment the patient becomes increasingly agitated and tachycardic with hypoxia. On examination the right side of the chest is hyperresonant with no audible breath sounds and the patient's trachea is deviated markedly to the left. What is the most appropriate next step?

A. Order an urgent chest X-ray
B. Insert a chest drain
C. Complete your initial assessment fully before initiating any further treatment
D. Insert a cannula into the mid clavicular line, second intercostal space on the right side
E. Insert a cannula into the mid clavicular line, second intercostal space on the left side

67. You are a GP FY2. A 20-year-old male with asthma presents asking for the seasonal flu vaccine. You are happy to give the patient the vaccine due to his long term respiratory disease. Which of the following patients would not routinely be recommended to have the seasonal flu vaccination?

    A. A 28-year-old pregnant patient who is in the third trimester
    B. A 66-year-old patient with no major medical problems
    C. A 32-year-old with Diabetes Mellitus
    D. A 22-year-old pregnant patient who is in the first trimester
    E. A 60-year-old patient with no major medical problems

68. A 40-year-old male who suffers from severe rheumatoid arthritis is struggling to conceive with his wife. The patient is referred to a fertility clinic where both he and his wife are assessed. The cause of the couple's infertility is found to be the patient's oligospermia. Which of the following medications is the likely cause?

    A. Cyclosporin
    B. Methotrexate
    C. Gold
    D. Sulfasalazine
    E. Azathioprine

69. A 60-year-old female patient is found to have a hyperdynamic apex beat on examination and on auscultation of the praecordium there is an early diastolic murmur which is accentuated by expiration. An echocardiogram confirms the diagnosis of aortic regurgitation. Which of the following physical signs is **not** associated with aortic regurgitation?

    A. Collapsing pulse
    B. Prominent carotid pulsation
    C. Quincke's sign
    D. Malar flush
    E. Wide pulse pressure

70, 71, 72. Regarding cranial nerves:

    A. Cranial nerve I
    B. Cranial nerve II
    C. Cranial nerve III
    D. Cranial nerve IV
    E. Cranial nerve V
    F. Cranial nerve VI
    G. Cranial nerve VII
    H. Cranial nerve VIII

For each of the following scenarios choose the cranial nerve from the options above which is most likely to be affected. Each option can be used once, more than once, or not at all.

70.   A 55 year-old patient, with a history of gradual onset of left sided facial droop, presents. She now has complete paralysis of the left side of her face which is causing some drooling from the corner of her mouth and dryness of her left eye. When asked to raise her eyebrows she is unable to raise her left eyebrow.

71. A 60-year-old male patient with poorly controlled diabetes presents with double vision with associated frontal headache. On examination the patient is unable to abduct his right eye.

72.   A 50-year-old male patient presents with severe facial pain. He has had several episodes of excruciating pain affecting the right side of his face. Each attack lasts for 1 or 2 minutes. He states that these attacks are often precipitated by shaving his face or brushing his teeth. On one occasion a cold gust of wind caused an episode of the pain.

73.   A 52-year-old patient has been suffering with symptoms of the menopause for several months and haematological tests have confirmed the diagnosis. She is keen to start hormone replacement therapy (HRT) because the symptoms are impacting greatly on her life. Before starting the treatment she wants to discuss the risks and potential benefits of the treatment. The risk of which of the following is reduced by taking HRT?

A.   Breast cancer
B.   Deep vein thrombosis
C.   Gallbladder disease
D.   Stroke
E.   Osteoporosis

74.   A 32-year-old woman presents because she is concerned about vaginal discharge. Over recent weeks she has developed grey vaginal discharge which is associated with a strong "fish-like" smell. You suspect bacterial vaginosis. What is the most appropriate treatment?

A.   Doxycycline
B.   Regular vaginal douching
C.   Benzylpenicillin
D.   Metronidazole
E.   Ceftriaxone

75. A 16-year-old boy presents with his mother. He has been unwell for a few days with headache and a temperature. He has now developed bilateral parotid swelling. He has no past medical history of note but he has not had any of his childhood vaccinations. You suspect he has developed mumps. Accordingly, because it is a notifiable disease, you notify the Health Protection Agency (HPA). Which of the following is **not** a notifiable disease?

    A. Meningococcal septicaemia
    B. Tuberculosis
    C. Measles
    D. Whooping cough
    E. Syphilis

76. A 28-year-old female who is 30 weeks pregnant, presents with sudden onset abdominal pain and decreased foetal movements. On examination she has a hard uterus and is in severe pain. There is no obvious vaginal discharge. The patient is tachycardic and hypotensive and despite several efforts you cannot locate a foetal heartbeat. What is the most likely diagnosis?

    A. Placenta praevia
    B. Appendicitis
    C. Placenta accreta
    D. Placental abruption
    E. Placenta increta

77, 78, 79. Regarding causative organisms:

    A. *Escherichia coli*
    B. *Staphylococcus saprophyticus*
    C. *Streptococcus viridans*
    D. *Chlamydia pneumoniae*
    E. *Mycoplasma pneumoniae*
    F. *Pseudomonas aeruginosa*
    G. *Legionella pneumophila*

For each of the following scenarios choose the most common causative organism from the list above. Each option may be used once, more than once, or not at all.

77. A 60-year-old female patient presents with dysuria, frequency and urgency. She is diagnosed with a urinary tract infection.

78. A 60-year-old patient presents acutely with pyrexia of unknown origin. After multiple investigations the patient is diagnosed with bacterial endocarditis.

79. A 60-year-old man presents with a week history of a painful right ear. The ear hurts to touch and there has been some offensive discharge. Examination of the ear reveals a severely inflamed external auditory canal. You suspect a case of acute otitis externa.

80. A 20-year-old patient with asthma presents with worsening asthma control. Since being diagnosed a year ago the patient has had relatively good control of his symptoms by using a starting dose of inhaled steroid and salbutamol inhaler as required. However, over recent months, despite good adherence to treatment and correct technique, his symptoms have gradually worsened. What would be the most appropriate next step in his management?

    A. Add in long acting beta agonist (LABA)
    B. Increase dose of inhaled steroid
    C. Add in leukotriene receptor antagonist
    D. Add in regular oral steroid
    E. Add in theophylline

81. A 65-year-old female patient presents in a distressed state. Recently she has started to pass small amounts of urine whenever she strains or coughs. This has started to affect her confidence and she is very distressed by the symptoms. She is otherwise well and her only past medical history is of three normal vaginal deliveries more than 30 years ago. What is the most likely diagnosis?

    A. Functional incontinence
    B. Stress incontinence
    C. Urge incontinence
    D. Urinary tract infection
    E. Overflow incontinence

82, 83, 84. Regarding lumps in the neck:

    A. Laryngeal carcinoma
    B. Carotid body tumour
    C. Thyroglossal cyst
    D. Pharyngeal pouch
    E. Pleomorphic adenoma
    F. Goitre
    G. Papillary adenocarcinoma
    H. Branchial cyst

For each of the following scenarios choose the most likely diagnosis from the list above. Each option may be used once, more than once, or not at all.

82. A 55-year-old man presents with a slow-growing mass in the anterior triangle of the neck. On examination the mass is pulsatile and a bruit is felt.

83. A 23-year-old student presents with an enlarging lump in the anterior triangle of his neck. The painless, fluctuant mass arises on the anterior aspect of the sternocleidomastoid muscle and does not move on protrusion of the tongue or on swallowing.

84. A 40-year-old woman presents with a neck lump. She also complains of feeling hot all of the time and has lost some weight recently. On examination there is a smooth diffuse and symmetrical mass in the anterior aspect of the neck. You note also that she has exophthalmos.

85. A concerned mother presents with her 6-month-old child who has recently become unwell. The child has been vomiting and is clearly in some abdominal discomfort. His mother explains that he has passed several stools which are red and "jelly-like". What is the most likely diagnosis?

A. Pyloric stenosis
B. Mesenteric adenitis
C. Biliary atresia
D. Appendicitis
E. Intussusception

86. Which of the following topical steroids is the most potent?

A. Dermovate
B. Eumovate
C. Elocon
D. Hydocortisone 1%
E. Betnovate

87. A 27-year-old student presents to you in general practice to discuss his recent hospital admission. He was admitted following his first unprovoked seizure. So far all investigations have been normal and he is awaiting follow up from the neurology department. How long after his first unprovoked epileptic seizure will this patient be able to drive his car again?

A. Minimum of 1 month
B. Minimum of 2 month
C. Minimum of 6 months
D. Minimum of 12 months
E. Minimum of 24 months

88. A 55-year-old man presents to you in primary care for a routine blood pressure check. His blood pressure is slightly high and while discussing non-pharmacological management you suggest that reducing his alcohol intake might be a worthwhile step. What is the current recommended guidance on male alcohol intake in the UK?

A. No more than 14 units of alcohol per week
B. No more than 17 units of alcohol per week
C. No more than 19 units of alcohol per week
D. No more than 21 units of alcohol per week
E. No more than 23 units of alcohol per week

89. A 35-year-old badminton player presents to A&E unable to weight-bear after injuring himself while jumping during a match. He felt a sudden pain at the back of his right ankle and heard an audible "snap". On examination he is in pain and unable to fully plantar-flex his right foot. You suspect he may have ruptured his Achilles tendon. Which of the following tests might help you in your clinical assessment?

A. Finkelstein's test
B. Allen's test
C. Ortolani test
D. Simmonds' test
E. Hess test

90. A 19-year-old female patient presents during her first pregnancy. Some routine blood tests and measurements are performed. Regarding normal physiological changes in pregnancy, which one of the following decreases during normal pregnancy?

A. Cardiac output
B. Total blood volume
C. White blood count
D. Haemoglobin concentration
E. Glomerular filtration rate

91. A 25-year-old female patient presents for a routine appointment. You notice incidentally that she has marked staining of her teeth which, she explains, is long standing and is due to an antibiotic she was prescribed when she was a child. Which of the following should **not** be prescribed to children due to the risk of dental staining?

   A. Tetracycline
   B. Erythromycin
   C. Meropenem
   D. Clarithromycin
   E. Metronidazole

92. A 3-year-old boy presents with his parents who are very anxious. He is normally fit and well but recently has had several bouts of balanitis. His parents are concerned that when he passes urine the stream is poor and there is marked ballooning of the foreskin. On examination the opening of the prepuce is very small and the foreskin itself not retractable. What is the most likely diagnosis?

   A. Paraphimosis
   B. Phimosis
   C. Hypospadias
   D. Epispadias
   E. Priapism

93. A 25-year-old student presents with a history of back pain and lethargy. Over recent months he has developed severe lower back pain which is worst in the mornings and improves with movement. He has little past medical history of note apart from an isolated episode of iritis earlier in the year. What is the most likely diagnosis?

   A. Rheumatoid arthritis
   B. Ankylosing spondylitis
   C. Osteoarthritis
   D. Perthes' disease
   E. Spinal fracture

94. A 75-year-old patient has recently been started on a new medication for rheumatoid arthritis. She is distressed because she has started to develop excessive hair growth all over her body. Which of the following medications is the most likely cause for her symptom?

A. Azathioprine
B. Mycophenolate mofetil
C. Gold
D. Cyclosporin
E. Methotrexate

95. An 80-year-old female presents with multiple skin lesions all over her back. She finds them unsightly and would like to know what they are. She explains that they have been present for many years and have not changed recently. The lesions are raised brown spots which have a warty surface and have a "stuck on" appearance. What is the most likely diagnosis?

A. Basal cell carcinoma
B. Actinic keratosis
C. Bowen's disease
D. Malignant melanoma
E. Seborrhoeic keratosis

96. A 52-year-old woman presents with a lump in her groin. On examination the lump is smooth, non-tender and compressible. It transmits a cough impulse, disappears when the patient lies flat and has a noticeable blue tinge to it. What is the most likely diagnosis?

A. Saphena varix
B. Psoas abscess
C. Lymph node
D. Femoral artery aneurysm
E. Spigelian hernia

97. A 78-year-old patient who is taking warfarin for atrial fibrillation is found to have a markedly raised INR following a course of antibiotics. The haematologist advises a dose of vitamin K in order to reduce the INR. Which one of the following is not a vitamin K–dependent clotting factor?

A. II
B. VII
C. VIII
D. IX
E. X

98. A 20-year-old patient with type 1 diabetes presents acutely with vomiting and pyrexia. He has been unwell for a couple of days with a cough and began vomiting a few hours ago. His blood glucose measurement is 28 mmol/L and the pH on a venous blood sample is 7.1. Additionally, he has ketonuria. What is the most likely diagnosis?

A. Diabetic ketoacidosis
B. Hypoglycaemia
C. Insulin overdose
D. Simple hyperglycaemia
E. Hyperosmolar hyperglycaemic state

99. A 55-year-old estate agent is admitted acutely to hospital after suffering from a myocardial infarction. Driving is essential for his work and he would like to know how long it will be before he can drive again. For how long after suffering from a myocardial infarction should a patient abstain from driving?

A. No need to abstain
B. 2 weeks
C. 4 weeks
D. 2 months
E. 6 months

100. An 80-year-old female was found to have an isolated raised alkaline phosphatase with a normal calcium and phosphate level. She also had reduced hearing and developed symptoms of heart failure. After extensive investigations the patient was diagnosed with Paget's disease of the bone. Which of the following are patients with Paget's disease at increased risk of?

A. Lung cancer
B. Meningioma
C. Sarcoma
D. Lipoma
E. Squamous cell carcinoma

Chapter 5
Stage 3 explained

After the Stage 2 online exam, all of the candidates in the country are ranked according to their scores and this rank is used to allocate candidates to a selection centre. Allocation to a Stage 3 selection centre (within a deanery) is done according to the deanery preferences that you made during the Stage 1 online application. The candidates who ranked highest in the Stage 2 exam are offered Stage 3 places in their first choice deanery.

If you have not scored highly enough in Stage 2, and all of the places in your top choice deanery have already been allocated (to higher scoring candidates), then you will be offered a place in the next deanery that you have ranked which still has places remaining. *Figure 5.1* explains this more clearly than a long paragraph can. In previous years candidates have also been given details of their Stage 2 score at this point.

Selection Centre Allocation Examples

Example 1
During his Stage 1 online application Tim made the following preference with regards to deaneries:

1st London Recruitment
2nd Health Education East of England
3rd Health Education Kent, Surrey and Sussex

In the Stage 2 online exam Tim scored very highly and therefore when the NRO came to allocating selection centres for the Stage 3 assessment there were still spaces in the London Recruitment deanery. Hence, Tim will now receive an invitation to sit his Stage 3 assessment in London. This does not guarantee Tim a GP training post in London. He still needs to perform well in the Stage 3 interview.

Example 2

During her Stage 1 online application Amy made the following preference with regards to deaneries (the same as Tim):

1st *London Recruitment*
2nd *Health Education East of England*
3rd *Health Education Kent, Surrey and Sussex*

Amy did well in the Stage 2 online exam but did not rank at the very top of the Stage 2 exam scores. Unfortunately, when the NRO came to allocating Amy to a selection centre for the Stage 3 assessment there were no places left in the London deanery as they had already been filled by candidates who had scored more highly. There were, however, spaces available in the East of England deanery and therefore Amy was offered a Stage 3 selection centre place in this deanery. Like Tim, this does <u>not</u> guarantee Amy a GP training post in the East of England. However, it does mean that Amy <u>cannot</u> now get a training post in London.

Figure 5.1 – Examples of how selection centre places are allocated for the Stage 3 assessment

If none of your ranked deaneries has places left for Stage 3 then your application will cease at this point. While this is unlikely to happen, it is worth considering this when ranking your deanery preferences during your initial application.

As mentioned in *Chapter 3*, in recent years there has been as second round of applications which occur in March. This round, often called "round one re-advert", occurs when there are excess training posts available which have been unfilled during the first round of applications. The quantity and the geographical locations of the posts available in the "round one re-advert" vary from year to year. Applications for this round are open to new candidates, those who have shown sufficient evidence in Stage 2 but have not been allocated a deanery, and those who have not shown enough evidence.

In the latter case, applicants will need to re-sit the Stage 2 assessment. Importantly, due to there being fewer posts available during the round one re-advert, there are fewer Stage 3 assessment centres allocated for this process and therefore candidates may need to be prepared to travel quite some distance in order to be assessed. Some candidates, who want a specific deanery which is not available in the round one re-advert, may choose not to apply during this round of applications and instead may choose to reapply afresh the following November.

Allocation to a Stage 3 selection centre within a deanery does not guarantee a training post. Instead it confirms that you have been granted the opportunity to sit the next assessment in the application process.

Selection centres offer around 1.5 Stage 3 places for every training post vacancy available in the deanery; therefore there are more applicants sitting Stage 3 than there are available posts. This is done deliberately as some applicants will withdraw from the GP application process after Stage 3, as they might accept training posts in other specialties, or withdraw for personal reasons.

A very small minority will not score highly enough in the Stage 3 assessment to be offered a post. These applicants can reapply for a GP training post during the round one re-advert period in March. These candidates will have already satisfied both the Stage 1 criteria and the Stage 2 assessment requirements and therefore will not need to repeat these steps if they choose to reapply in March. They will of course need to re-attempt the Stage 3 examination.

Invitations to attend Stage 3 selection centres are sent out shortly after the Stage 2 exam. This will happen towards the end of January or the beginning of February. Candidates are notified via email and can book their place via the Oriel application system. Assessments normally take place in the first two weeks of February.

In addition to an invitation to attend the Stage 3 exam you will also usually be asked to indicate your geographical sub-preferences within the deanery to which you have been allocated. Each deanery has a different mechanism for allocating posts internally so it is worth taking the time to visit the deanery website to gain more information about the particular nuances of that deanery. Most will allocate posts according to the combined scores from Stage 2 and Stage 3 with the highest scoring candidates getting their highest preference. For further details on how your deanery operates and their reasoning for doing so, consult their individual website.

The format of the Stage 3 examination

The Stage 3 examination will take place over a number of days at a selection centre within your allocated deanery. It takes the format of an hour long examination split into a single 30 minute written prioritisation task and three simulated scenarios, each of which is 10 minutes long (*Figure 5.2*). The simulated patient/carer/colleague is played by an actor and an examiner also sits in the room to observe the consultation.

During the written station you will likely be in a room with around 20 other candidates. During the simulated stations you will be rotating through the stations with around two other candidates, with each of you taking it in turns to tackle one of the three scenarios.

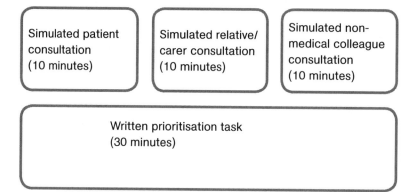

Figure 5.2 – The Stage 3 examination format

Where you start on the diagram will vary depending on your selection centre. However, it is worth bearing in mind that you will either do the written prioritisation task first, **or** the three scenarios (i.e. you would not be asked to do a clinical scenario, then the written task followed by a further two clinical scenarios). However, the order that you do the three simulated scenarios will be random and may not be in the order illustrated in *Figure 5.2*.

In each of the sections of this exam you will be judged by your ability to demonstrate sufficient evidence that you fulfil the qualities required in the ST1 personal specification (see *Appendix*). These can broadly be broken down into:

- Problem Solving

- Professionalism

- Empathy

- Communication Skills

This is not an exhaustive list, but it can be helpful to keep these in mind during Stage 3. If you are found to show insufficient evidence of any of these during the assessment then your application will not progress further.

What to expect on the day

Prior to the assessment day you will receive details from your allocated deanery about when and where to arrive and what to take with you on the day. It is crucial that you read these details carefully as the list is extensive and fail–

ure to present the required documents on the day may lead to a delay in your offer of employment as well as adding avoidable stress. Typically the sorts of documents required on the day include (but are not limited to):

- Photographic I.D.

- Details of immigration status

- Original GMC certificate

- Medical Degree certificate

- Evidence of Foundation Competency

- Evidence of current DBS/CRB

Details of what you should wear usually accompany the email. Typically you should dress smartly and in attire appropriate for the wards. On the day arrive in plenty of time and assume that there will be no refreshments provided. You will be greeted by deanery staff prior to the assessment and they will go through your documentation before explaining how the day will run. You will then sit your assessments and usually afterwards there is a group debriefing with a "question & answer" session with a member of deanery staff.

Tips on how to do well

The key to doing well in Stage 3 is good time management. It is therefore imperative to practise both the written and practical stations before the day. Ideally you should start practising for this exam as soon as you have finished Stage 2.

There is a multitude of ways to rehearse for this assessment and therefore it's worth spending a bit of time considering which methods you want to focus on. For the simulated scenario stations there is no practice better than teaming up with some like-minded friends and taking it in turns to be the candidate, actor and examiner. A full practice paper is provided in *Chapter 6*.

However you choose to rehearse the Stage 3 assessments, the onus must be on good time management. Below we consider the two components individually.

The written station

This station takes place as a 30 minute handwritten exam paper. The paper starts with a set of instructions followed by a scenario. The purpose of the scenario is to set the scene for the five options which follow it. You, as the candidate, must firstly rank the five actions/responses in the order in which you would prioritise them. Then in the five answer boxes provided, explain why you have prioritised particular tasks in the places that you have chosen and explain how you will go about tackling each one. You should only aim to talk about one task in each box and you should try to make several bullet points of explanation for each task. This is, perhaps, best illustrated with an example (*Figure 5.3*).

Written Prioritisation Task – Example 1

"You are an FY2 doctor on a busy surgical ward coming to the end of your 12 hour night shift. You have one hour left of your shift before you hand over to the day team"

You must prioritise the tasks below in the order in which you would action them.

You must:
1. *Rank the tasks appropriately*
2. *Explain why you have made these decisions and how you will complete the tasks*
3. *Reflect on this exercise*

You have 30 minutes to complete this task.

Any entries made outside of the answer boxes will not be marked
A. *A nurse from the ward calls to tell you that one of the surgical patients has developed severe central chest pain and is becoming sweaty and clammy.*
B. *The surgical registrar bleeps you to ask if you can write up tonight's dose of prophylactic heparin for a patient who was operated on in the early hours as she had forgotten to do it and she is now scrubbed in theatre.*
C. *Your partner has texted you asking you to call her urgently.*
D. *You see one of the nurses run past you in floods of tears and rush into the bathroom sobbing.*
E. *You have an abstract that needs completing and submitting to a prestigious international meeting. The deadline is in fifty minutes' time.*

Figure 5.3 – *Written Prioritisation Task – Example 1*

Following your prioritisation and explanation of the five options there is then a reflection exercise in which you must reflect on the challenges of the task and what you have learned. This usually takes the form of three structured questions.

Inevitably you will feel that you have lots to write about the task that you prioritise first. However, the marks for this part of the exam are split evenly between each of the five tasks. A good exam technique is to initially restrict yourself to a few bullet points in each box. Hence, even though you may have seven or even eight points for the first answer, you should move on and ensure you have sufficient entries in the subsequent boxes. By all means return to the first box to add further points if you finish in time, but your priority should be to make several points in all the boxes in the first instance.

Unlike the Professional Dilemmas in the Stage 2 exam there is much less onus on the order in which you prioritise these tasks. The justification for your order is the main thing being assessed. However, you may find it hard to justify ranking a medical emergency as the fifth most important task if the other options are clearly not as pressing. Additionally, time is very tight for this task and you will find yourself writing up until the last second. One of the biggest errors that you can make is deciding halfway through to change the order of prioritisation and therefore make a complete mess of the exam paper. A key piece of advice is therefore to take a minute or two at the start of the exam to decide on your order and then stick to it!

The scenario in *Figure 5.3* is fairly typical of what to expect, although as mentioned previously, scenarios in this part of the exam do not always involve clinical tasks. In this case I would have chosen the order A, C, E, D, B. The order that you select for this scenario may be different but, as discussed above, the marks for this task lie in the justification of your prioritisation. *Figure 5.4* shows an example justification for my first choice answer.

Example Prioritisation Answer

1st Option: **A**
- I have prioritised this option first as the patient may be suffering from a myocardial infarction which is a medical emergency and therefore will need urgent assessment.
- I would not be able to concentrate on the other tasks if I had not attended this patient first.
- While I was on the phone to the nurse I would ask her some more details so that I can be formulating a plan while on my way to the patient.
- I would request that she do a fresh set of observations and an ECG so that it is ready for my arrival.

Figure 5.4 – Example prioritisation answer

Figure 5.4 shows the types of things you could put down in the white box. There are clearly many more things you could say, but in order to complete the task you should move on and return if you have time. Generally issues regarding patient safety should be acted on early. It is also important to think of which other members of staff could help you in each situation (nurses, healthcare assistants, other doctors, receptionists). It helps to show problem solving ability and the capacity to delegate tasks. It is also important to consider if any of the tasks can wait until later, or if they could be handed over. These are important considerations as they show the ability to think conceptually and manage time effectively.

Figure 5.4 also illustrates the balance needed between justification and actions. The marks for these questions are split evenly between the two. In the example above the first two points justify why I have ranked this option first, followed by two points outlining the actions I have taken. It is important to include both justifications and actions in each box in order to ensure you get the most marks.

As for the other options in this scenario (*Figure 5.3*) you would need to justify why you had prioritised each. It would be reasonable to suggest that option C needed addressing next as it would undoubtedly distract you from the other tasks if you left it until later, and additionally it would likely be a quick task to complete (phoning/texting your partner back). Option E is also quite a distracting task and is time-dependent which adds an extra dimension. Clearly it should have been done earlier and therefore an interesting point to make as part of your answer might be:

"I would later reflect on why I had left this submission to the last minute to ensure that I could avoid recurrence of this problem in the future."

Option D is clearly an important event to review. It is a great opportunity to show empathy and sensitivity in your answer by suggesting that you would speak to the nurse about why she was upset and offer any help you could. It would be reasonable to suggest that option B was the least crucial task on the basis that the dose of heparin is a prophylactic evening dose and furthermore with handover only an hour away, it would be a very reasonable task to hand over unlike all of the other tasks. In the exam you would of course then be expected to reflect on what you found difficult and what you have learned from this task.

It is easy to see that the written prioritisation task is a challenging exercise in just 30 minutes. The key is clearly to practise these scenarios. By practising with a friend (ideally someone who is also doing the exam) you can bounce ideas off each other which can be helpful. Try to imagine the everyday scenarios that you deal with at work as real life prioritisation tasks and think how you would justify your prioritisation if you had to do so in the exam.

The simulated scenarios

The simulated scenarios will arguably be a more familiar assessment modality than the written prioritisation task as they are essentially an OSCE. Anyone who has come through the UK medical education system will be familiar with OSCEs, but they may be unfamiliar for overseas candidates. If you are unfamiliar with OSCEs than I would recommend you read one of the many OSCE books written for medical students and look at sample OSCE consultations online. As outlined above (*Figure 5.2*) there are three 10 minute long simulated scenarios: with a patient; a carer/relative; and a non-medical co-worker.

It's important to remember that this assessment is not testing your clinical knowledge, as this has been tested in Stage 2. It is instead testing you against the areas of the personal specification highlighted earlier. As a reminder, the key elements of this are:

- Problem Solving

- Professionalism

- Empathy

- Communication Skills

Therefore you will not be expected to take a history or examine the patient in the scenario. While you may need to briefly rule out any red flag symptoms (if the scenario requires it), you should instead concentrate on your communication skills and the consultation as a whole.

The location of selection centres varies wildly with some taking place in conference centres and some in the corporate boxes of a local sports stadium. Irrespective of the venue the arrangements for the day will be vaguely similar. You will be called into a room where there will usually be two chairs, a table and an examiner. The examiners are under strict instructions to stay silent throughout the whole process, so do not be put off if they sit there stony-faced throughout.

When requested to do so you can turn over the piece of paper on the desk. Your 10 minutes have started at this point. Read the instructions carefully and take a moment to think the scenario through before getting up and calling the actor into the room. You must remember to call the actor in otherwise you will score no points: remember the examiner is duty bound to say nothing and therefore cannot help you.

It is likely that as you are at the level of an FY2 or above you will be inherently good at consultations in this manner. Some useful hints however include:

General tips

- After reading the candidate instructions think the scenario through for a moment before calling the actor in.

- Keep an open mind about the arrangement of the room and do not be afraid to move the chairs if you feel it will aid your consultation.

- Start with open questions. The actor is likely to have an opening line or phrase to use, so give them a chance to help you by allowing them to answer open questions initially.

- Make sure you listen to the actor as they are telling you which way the consultation should go. Importantly, show the examiner that you are actively listening with your body language.

- Look for clues and hints. There is often a subplot to the scenario and the actor will be trying to give you clues so look out for these.

- In virtually all scenarios it is useful to explore the actor's Ideas, Concerns and Expectations (ICE) (*Figure 5.5*).

- Try to aim to come up with a shared plan of how you will tackle the issues raised. Work through the problem together.

- Additionally, consider in each scenario if you can arrange a follow up meeting. For example, if you have agreed a plan with a co-worker to help with a problem they have been having, it might be nice to arrange to meet up in a week to see if things have improved.

- It's really useful to summarise what you have talked about at the end of the consultation as it helps bring the consultation to a close.

- Try to keep an eye on the time but don't get worried if you finish early or if you don't finish in time as it gives no indication of the success of the station.

- Try not to let the previous station affect the next station (either positively or negatively).

- It is also important to recognise your own limitations and to seek senior help if required.

Ideas, Concerns and Expectations

Ideas, Concerns and Expectations, (often shortened to the mnemonic 'ICE'), is a tool used to help gather information during a consultation. It is particularly useful in the Stage 3 examination because it can help to ensure that you cover important points and explore any underlying issues that are not immediately apparent.

Ideas – Explore what the patient thinks is happening. In many cases the patient will have a preconceived idea of what the problem is.

Concerns – Is there anything in particular that the patient is worried about? Why are they anxious about this issue? This line of questioning is often useful in uncovering hidden issues.

Expectations – It can be really important to establish the patient's expectations of a consultation early on so that these can be managed appropriately. This line of questioning can be helpful in ensuring that the patient is satisfied with the consultation.

Figure 5.5 – Ideas, Concerns and Expectations

Simulated patient consultation

- Remember, this is not really a test of your medical knowledge (as this has already been assessed in Stage 2). The scenario will have, instead, been designed to test your consultation skills.

- Make sure you listen to the actor as they are telling you which way the consultation should go.

- Importantly, show the examiner that you are actively listening with your body language.

- Avoid the temptation to make the conversation too clinical. If you end up taking a history in the patient station you have gone wrong as the scenario will have been designed to test your consultation skills. An exception to this might be to briefly touch on "red flag" symptoms if the scenario demands it.

- It's really important to show empathy throughout.

- Good communication skills are crucial, but so is checking understanding, so make sure you allow time to check that the actor has understood what you've discussed.

- If the scenario demands it make sure you consider risk. If it's a patient who is struggling with their mood it is reasonable to ask about suicidal ideas for example.

Simulated relative/carer consultation

- As with the simulated patient scenario, there is often a hidden agenda, so keep this in mind.

- Some scenarios may involve an angry relative (or patient). Try to calm the situation down so that you can have a meaningful dialogue.

- Consider offering suitable resources to the relative/carer where they can find further information, for example a leaflet or website.

- Again, ensure that the relative/carer has understood what you have discussed and allow them to ask any questions they may have.

Simulated non-medical colleague consultation

- Try to elicit if the person has any support network available to them such as friends and family who might be able to help in the current situation.

- If appropriate to the scenario consider exploring the psychosocial impact of what is going on. For example, whether the problem affecting their sleep, or if are they drinking more than usual to help them cope. This is also true of the patient based scenario.

- While it's important to delegate work it can also be crucial to show that you can personally take responsibility for tasks too.

- Try to remember that you are talking to a colleague and avoid turning the consultation into a patient–like consultation. This is easier said than done.

Importantly, try to keep an eye on the time but don't get worried if you finish early, or if you don't finish in time as it gives no indication of the success of the station. Try not to let the previous station affect the next station and try if you can to smile and be relaxed. There is no substitute for practice however, so we have provided a full Stage 3 example paper with answers and discussions (*Chapter 6 – Stage 3 Practice Paper*).

REMEMBER!

- Make sure you have all of your documents in order so as to avoid unnecessary added stress on the day.
- Practise, Practise, Practise, – ideally with a friend who is also doing the exam.
- Keep an eye on the time throughout the exam.
- Don't let the previous station affect the current station.
- Smile and try to look confident and relaxed.

Chapter 6
Stage 3 practice paper

This exam is made up of two parts: a 30 minute written prioritisation task and three 10 minute simulated clinical scenarios. In order to make the most of this practice examination you should find a partner to act as the patient, carer/relative, co-worker in the scenarios. It does not matter which order you attempt the clinical scenarios or the written task. The whole exam should last 60 minutes.

Answers and explanations can be found in the answer section at the end of the book.

Clinical Scenario 1 *(10 minutes)*

You are an FY2 doctor working in the Accident and Emergency department. You are asked to see 20-year-old Katie Smith who wants to self-discharge. She has presented with abdominal pain and the consultant has decided that she needs admission for blood tests and an ultrasound scan as she may have appendicitis.

Clinical Scenario 1 – Information for the Simulated Patient

Your mood: Anxious

Background: You are 20 year old Katie Smith and you have come to A&E because you have tummy pain.

- You have been told by the consultant that you need to stay for blood tests and a 'scan' of your tummy as you might have appendicitis and this has made you very anxious.
- Although you are in pain you want to self-discharge from hospital because you don't want to be admitted.
- You are not worried about the blood tests or scan but you are worried about the possibility that you might need an operation. You are worried about the anaesthetic and that you might not "wake up" and you are also concerned that there might be complications to the surgery itself.
- You would feel a bit better if your mum could come and join you from home to hold your hand. You are hoping that the doctor will reassure you.
- You will be happy to stay if the doctor offers you sufficient reassurance.

Information to reveal only if asked:
If asked about why you are worried you should explain that your grandfather died a few months ago in this hospital because of complications following surgery to repair an aneurysm in his tummy and this is playing on your mind.

Clinical Scenario 2

Clinical Scenario 2 – Information for the Candidate

- You should read these instructions carefully.
- Read the scenario below in full and then call the simulated co-worker into the room.
- The examiner has been instructed not to speak under any circumstances.
- You have 10 minutes for this station. This includes the time taken to read the scenario.

You are an FY2 doctor on the Surgical Assessment Unit (SAU) when Wendy Collins, the ward clerk, asks if she can speak to you.

Clinical Scenario 2 – Information for the Simulated Co-Worker

Your mood: Upset

Background: You are Wendy Collins a 55-year-old ward clerk on the Surgical Assessment Unit (SAU).

- You have worked on SAU for 10 years and enjoy your work. You work two and a half days per week and your colleague Sally works the other two and a half days. Recently Sally has been off sick and you have been asked to cover her shifts.
- Initially you were happy to do so as you needed the extra money and you understood it would be for a maximum of 2 weeks. That was 6 weeks ago and there is no sign of Sally returning to work. Despite this your manager is still expecting you to cover her shifts and did not respond well when you explained that you are finding the extra work so stressful. You are scared about discussing the issue further with your manager as a result.
- One of the reasons you are finding it so stressful is that your only daughter, who is a 25-year-old single mum, has a new baby and you previously tried to spend the two and half days a week that you were not working by helping her.
- You live at home with your husband who works nights at a local factory. You feel like you haven't seen him properly for weeks because you are now working all day every day and he is working nights.
- You are finding it difficult to sleep because you lie awake at night worrying about the situation.
- You drink about a bottle of wine per week and don't smoke. Your drinking hasn't increased recently and you are otherwise well.
- You have asked to speak to this doctor as you have a good working relationship and wonder if they have any ideas of how you could improve your situation.

Information to reveal only if asked:
Despite feeling upset and anxious, your mood is fine and you have no suicidal thoughts.

Clinical Scenario 3

Clinical Scenario 3 – Information for the Candidate

- You should read these instructions carefully.
- Read the scenario below in full and then when you are ready call the simulated relative/carer into the room.
- The examiner has been instructed not to speak under any circumstances.
- You have 10 minutes for this station. This includes the time taken to read the scenario.

You are an FY2 doctor on a general medical ward. The daughter of Mrs Smith has asked to speak to you. Mrs Smith, who is 89-years-old, was initially admitted with a urinary tract infection which has been successfully treated. However the patient's family have raised concerns about her memory and as part of her comprehensive assessment Mrs Smith has been diagnosed with dementia (Alzheimer's type). Mrs Smith's daughter, Mary, is concerned about her mother being discharged home alone in her current state.

You have permission to discuss Mrs Smith's case with her daughter.

Clinical Scenario 3 – Information for the Simulated Relative

Your mood: Angry

Background: You are Mary and your mother (Mrs. Smith) was initially admitted with urine infection which has been treated. You raised concerns with the team that your mum's memory has worsened over the last 6 months and after further assessment she has been diagnosed with Alzheimer's dementia.

- You are concerned and angry because you feel as though the medical team are going to send your mum home alone without adequate support. You are worried about what the future holds for your mum and don't think she can cope at home alone.
- You don't know much about Alzheimer's disease but you recently read in a tabloid newspaper that stem cell treatment could be adapted to treat the condition and you expect that this could offer your mum some hope.

Information to reveal only if asked directly:
You are really concerned about who would pay for any carers as your mother doesn't have any savings and you and your husband will not be able to cover the cost of carers.

Written Prioritisation Task

- You have 30 minutes to complete this task.
- Carefully read the scenario below in full and then read the five tasks which follow. In the answer boxes provided prioritise the tasks in the order in which you would complete them and in each box justify why you have placed that task in that box.
- Finally you must complete the reflection exercise on the final page by answering the questions provided.
- Only answers that are within the boxes will be marked.

You are an FY2 working on the Surgical Assessment Unit (SAU). You are a few hours into your shift and you have the following tasks to complete. Please prioritise these in the order you would do them.

A. *The ward clerk asks you to complete discharge summaries for four patients who were discharged yesterday.*

B. *A healthcare assistant approaches you to discuss your registrar who she feels has been making derogatory comments about the care she is providing to patients.*

C. *A staff nurse informs you that the relative of a patient who has developed a postoperative complication wants to speak to you about making a formal complaint. The relative is very angry.*

D. *A patient is due to have surgery this afternoon and has some questions.*

E. *Your partner has sent you a text message asking you to call her as soon as possible.*

Written Prioritisation Task – Answer Boxes

1st Task:

2nd Task:

3rd Task:

4th Task:

5th Task:

Written Prioritisation Task – Reflection Exercise

What aspect of this task did you find the hardest?

What did you do well?

What could you have done better?

Chapter 7
Stage 4 and beyond

Congratulations on reaching this point! It is now mid-February and you are coming to the end of a long process which began in November. All the hard work is done and it is now a case of waiting. You have made it to Stage 4 in the application process which covers the allocation of posts by the deanery and acceptance by the candidates.

Offers for posts are usually released towards the end of February. If successful you will be offered a post for your first choice sub-preference within the deanery in which you sat your Stage 3 assessment (e.g. Bristol, within the Health Education South West Deanery).

Once offers are made via the online Oriel system you have only 48 hours to make a decision about what you would like to do. **This is a crucial point in the whole process**. You must keep your eyes fixed on your emails and your Oriel account around the date of the offer release. Failure to respond to an offer within 48 hours will lead to your offer being withdrawn and all of your hard work will have been in vain! Importantly the 48 hours **includes** weekends and bank holidays so you really must act quickly. This therefore means that, if you are due to be hiking in the Himalayas or exploring deepest Siberia, you must plan ahead and make provisions for responding to any offers that you might receive.

After receiving an offer you will have three options via the online Oriel system:

1. You can **accept** the offer. This is where the whole process ends and you can then relax knowing that your GP VTS post is secured. See below for the possibility of "upgrades." If you accept your GP training post you will automatically decline offers from any other specialties you have applied for.

2. You can **hold** the offer. This will be because you are still waiting to hear from another specialty application that you have made. You will be able to hold the offer up until a specific date (usually in mid-March). Failure to make a

decision about the offer before this deadline has passed will lead to the offer being automatically withdrawn. So while it buys you some time to hear from other specialties, you must still remember to make a decision to accept or decline the offer before the deadline. You can only hold one offer at a time. So if you have applied to more than one specialty you must carefully consult the details on the Oriel website about the consequences of your actions before doing anything. It would be easy to accidentally decline a post if you are not careful!

3. You can **decline** the offer. By doing this you are confirming that you do not wish to accept the post or any other upgrades. At this point your application ceases and you will have no training post.

The added component to the above options is the option to accept the post and "opt in for upgrades." This essentially applies when you have been successful in being offered a post in your preferred deanery but not at your preferred sub-preference within that deanery. Using the Health Education South West deanery as an example, "Candidate A" may have been offered a three year GP VTS post in Swindon which was her second choice when she ranked her sub-preferences within the deanery (Bristol being her top choice). "Candidate A" can accept the post at Swindon, and choose the option to "opt in for upgrades." This essentially means that if a place comes up in Bristol she would prefer that. It is perhaps easy to see why a place might become available. Candidates can apply for several specialties and therefore someone who might prefer an alternative specialty training post may decline the GP VTS post they have also been offered in Bristol – thus there would now be an unallocated post in Bristol. The allocation of these upgrades is done according to candidates' ranking within the deanery. There can be huge movement in some deaneries so it is worth considering this option if you would prefer one of your more highly ranked options. It's important to note that these upgrades will be automatic, so if you do opt in you will have no further say in where you end up as the system will continue to upgrade you as posts become available. Equally, if "Candidate A" accepts the post in Swindon and "opts for upgrades" and no "upgrades" become available, or she doesn't rank highly enough to gain one of the newly vacant Bristol posts, she must take the post in Swindon.

Each deanery takes different things into consideration when allocating rotations. "Opting for upgrades" could, in theory mean that you get a post in a more desired hospital, but may mean that you do not get the rotations you desire. This could occur if you have been "upgraded" from being one of the highest ranked candidates in an unpopular sub-preference, to being one of the lowest ranked candidates in a popular sub-preference. Therefore it is worth checking with your deanery of choice how these allocations are made.

If you are deemed appointable following Stage 3 (i.e. your performance met all the required criteria) but there are no more posts available in the deanery in which you were interviewed (because they have been allocated to candidates with higher overall scores) you will be considered for any posts in that deanery which are declined. Following this, if no posts are available in that deanery, you will be considered for remaining available posts in the other deaneries that you have ranked.

A small number of posts will remain unfilled despite the comprehensive clearing process outlined above. These posts will be offered during the "round one re-advert" process (mentioned in *Chapters 3 and 5*). This process also consists of Stages 1, 2, 3 and 4 and is open to both new candidates and those who have failed to progress through the full GP application process. Usually this occurs in March but dates for these applications vary so consult the NRO website for details.

Having accepted your GP training post the NRO will then contact the referees you provided in Stage 1. It is advisable to contact them yourself too in order to prompt them to complete their references in a timely manner as this must be done prior to formally being offered a post by your deanery.

At this stage you can expect to be contacted by the deanery directly who will give you information about forms you must complete, documents you must provide and details of your contract. You will also be offered the opportunity to rank the specific job rotations in your hospitals at a local level. Therefore you will not know which jobs you are doing within your training programme until the late spring/early summer. Finally, you will be asked to register with the Royal College of General Practitioners (RCGP) in order to receive your e-portfolio.

So after months of form filling, revision, practice and examinations you have reached the conclusion of the GP application process and the start of your journey to becoming a GP!

"This is not the end. It is not even the beginning of the end. But it is, perhaps, the end of the beginning"

– Winston Churchill

Answers to questions
Stage 2 practice paper answers and discussions

Professional Dilemma answers and discussions

1. **Correct Answer: A, C, E, B, D**

The first line action should be to speak directly to your registrar about this issue (option A). However, you should involve your consultant (option C) in the discussion irrespective of the outcome of option A. It is important that your consultant is aware of this issue as he/she is ultimately responsible for the care carried out by the team. Option E is a very reasonable step to take and should be ranked next. While option B may need to be taken at some stage, it should only be taken after options A, C and E have been thoroughly explored. You must act on your suspicions in this scenario as patient safety is at stake which is why option D is the least appropriate answer.

2. **Correct Answer: B, D, C, E, A**

This question is not only about confidentiality but also integrity. You should take responsibility for your error and therefore option B is the most appropriate answer. However, option D is a close second as it is important not to further exacerbate the situation. Option C is a wise choice as your consultant may be able to give you guidance on how best to manage the situation. Option E, while being an important point, doesn't solve the issue in the short term and therefore is ranked second last. Option A is the least appropriate as it shows lack of integrity.

3. **Correct Answer: D, C, A, E, B**

This situation is tricky because of the patient's occupation. However tempting it may be, you should not manage her injury differently because of this. It is important to discuss her ideas and concerns (option D) about the injury and subsequently to explain why you feel an X-ray is not indicated (option C). Good advice (option A) is still important and it shouldn't be assumed that just because she is an orthopaedic sister that she will know exactly how to manage her own ankle injury. Option E is important also because of this. Option B is the least appropriate option because it goes against your clinical judgment and would be an unnecessary investigation.

4. **Correct Answer: B, C, E, D, A**

Option B is the most appropriate choice. It is important that the patient's care does not suffer due to the staffing level and you are not currently busy with another clinical task. It will also help improve the feeling of teamwork between you and the nurse. Option C may help to highlight the issue to the hospital's management and therefore may reduce the chance of this problem arising again. Option E is worthwhile, although it does not help the immediate issue. Option D and A both fail to show evidence of your ability to work in a team and therefore are ranked last. Option A is clearly less appropriate than option D.

5. **Correct Answer: E, D, C, A, B**

The most appropriate steps initially in this situation would be to ask why the nurses disagreed with the management plan (option E) and then to explain the rationale behind it (option D). To make a complaint to the sister in charge (option C) or to report them to their governing body (option A) would likely inflame the situation, and in the latter case be disproportionate. Option B would undermine your consultant's clinical judgment and would therefore be the most inappropriate option.

6. **Correct Answer: D, C, A, E, B**

You cannot, as an FY2 doctor, consent the patient for surgery and therefore option D is the most appropriate answer. Option C shows a willingness to learn and is the next most appropriate answer. It is reasonable to then address the issues raised in option A. Reporting the registrar to the GMC would be a very disproportionate action at this stage. It would be more appropriate to talk to the registrar directly or to discuss the situation with your consultant but, as these are not options in this scenario, option E should be ranked fourth. Option B is wholly inappropriate and must be last.

7. **Correct Answer: D, B, C, A, E**

This scenario is all about patient safety. The most important thing is to ensure no harm comes of this error which is why option D is the most important. Option B ensures that the patient has the correct treatment for their infection and should be next. Option C should be next as your supervisor will need to know about the issue and will be able to guide you on the correct processes to follow from here. Option A therefore is the next most appropriate in order to learn and reflect from the situation. Option E is the least appropriate, as the aim of this scenario is to do no harm and by leaving the task until the end of clinic the patient in question may have already taken the antibiotic with potentially catastrophic consequences.

8. **Correct Answer: C, D, E, B, A**

Option C is the best course of action. If you opted not to mention the issues in question you would not give the registrar any opportunity to improve.

Option D is worthwhile as it may allow you to improve your own prac-tice. You should complete the form and therefore option E is preferential to option B. Option A would be unprofessional and is therefore ranked last.

9. **Correct Answer: A, D**

This has the potential to be a medical emergency and therefore you should attend the patient immediately. Option A is better than option D as you will have more information on arrival if you ask for an ECG over the phone. Any option which does not involve immediately attending the patient is poten-tially unsafe (options B, E and C).

10. **Correct Answer: C, D**

Option C is important. This is a difficult moral situation and you should speak to your senior for guidance. Option D is crucial. You are entitled to your views but it is important that the patient's care is unaffected. This could take the form of facilitating a consultation with another colleague who doesn't share your objections. Both options B and A are inappropriate options as they are both highly unprofessional. Option E is also inappropri-ate. If you have a conscientious objection to a procedure you should not feel forced into acting against your objection when there are alternative options available to you.

11. **Correct Answer: A, D, E**

The GMC guidance on such situations is clear. It states that doctors must help in an emergency, but must also act safely and within their competency level. Therefore options A, D and E are the most appropriate answers. Option B, which you may have chosen, is unsafe and therefore not correct.

12. **Correct Answer: A, C, E, D, B**

The priority here must be to put matters right by first ordering the correct scan (option A) and then apologising to Mr Smith for the error (option C). You should inform your supervising consultant next (option E) and then fill out the appropriate incident form (option D). To not tell Mr Smith of the error (option B) would be completely inappropriate regardless of whether the scan was normal or not.

13. **Correct Answer: A, C**

This question is about confidentiality and impartiality. Clearly you cannot divulge what the patient has said to you in confidence, to his mother (option C). It is reasonable to suggest that there are many causes of chest pain (option A) as, at this point, we have no idea if his chest pain has been caused by his drug taking or not. Options B, D, E and G are all inappropriate as they all involve breach of patient confidentiality. Option F is entirely inappropriate. Whatever your personal views on drug use, you should not allow them to affect your professional decision making.

14. **Correct Answer: C, E**

The GMC provides guidance regarding social media and it is well worth a read. In this situation, it would be most appropriate to consult this guidance (option E) and to discuss the case with your supervisor (option C). In this situation it would be unwise to contact the patient via the social media website (options A and B). Likewise, you should seek guidance before contacting the patient by phone (option D). It would be unwise to just ignore the message (option F) as it is an issue which needs addressing to ensure that it doesn't happen again.

15. **Correct Answer: B, C, D, E, A**

By simply apologising you may be able to defuse the situation yourself (option B), however if this fails the presence of one of the regular senior doctors may help the situation (option C). You should not obstruct the patient if they want to make a complaint (option D). The scenario clearly states that this is the third such occasion this week in which you have ended up running late so option E is likely to be of benefit, although it won't solve the immediate problem of the angry patient in your room. Option A is the least appropriate as it may inflame the situation further.

16. **Correct Answer: C, D, A, E, B**

Option C would be the best course of action initially. A polite conversation with your registrar might be enough to solve the issue. It would not be unreasonable to seek advice from your consultant about this issue, but clearly you should give your registrar an opportunity to know about the issue first and therefore option D is placed after option C. Option A may come across as unhelpful and may damage your relationship with the nurse, but as a course of action it is not entirely unreasonable if you make this point politely. Option E is a very disproportionate action to take. Your registrar is new to the hospital, this is seemingly the first time this has happened, and this was her first unsupervised list. With this in mind, to report this isolated incident to the GMC would be heavy-handed and more inappropriate than the other options available. Option B is downright dishonest. It does not help in the solving of the issue and may damage your own relationship with the nurse.

17. **Correct Answer: B, E, A, C, D**

Clearly the most appropriate answer here is to arrange a suitable time with your consultant to complete the required assessment in the proper manner (option B). Option E is the next most appropriate as it will mean that you complete the assessments appropriately. It would be preferable for your consultant to sign you off rather than a registrar from a different specialty as the registrar is likely to have their own foundation doctor's assessments to complete. Option A is a very worthwhile exercise but it in no way tackles the current issue of needing to complete your assessments. Option C is a poor option as it shows no commitment to completing the required assessments and may lead to you failing your end of year assessments. Option D is completely inappropriate and dishonest and could lead to severe disciplinary action and must be ranked last.

18. **Correct Answer: C, D, A, E, B**

The GMC has recently updated its guidance on doctors' use of social media. It sets out clear advice on what is and what is not acceptable on social media. The priority here should be to remove the posts in question from the social media site as soon as possible and therefore option C is the most appropriate. Option D should be next as clearly your colleague needs more information about the GMC guidance. Option A is appropriate as this issue should ideally be dealt with locally before being passed to a national level (option E). Option B is the worst option as it essentially makes you complicit in the inappropriate behaviour of your colleague.

19. **Correct Answer: B, E**

The GMC give clear guidance about this very scenario. Doctors must not encourage patients to give gifts to them or other organisations (options C and D). The GMC do not say that you cannot accept such gifts but they do state that any acceptance of gifts must not affect the doctor–patient relationship (option F). Most practices will have a policy regarding this situation. In this case seeking advice from your supervisor (option B) is a wise course of action. As you don't know the practice policy, accepting the gift (option E) would be appropriate as to not do so, or to rebuff the patient, may damage your relationship (option A).

20. **Correct Answer: B, E, C, A, D**

It is the driver's responsibility to inform the DVLA of his seizure. However, the doctor must make every effort to reiterate this to the patient if they do not do so (option B). If the patient refuses to accept this advice then the doctor should advise a second opinion (but instruct the patient not to drive in the meantime) (option E). The doctor, having tried at length to persuade the patient to inform the DVLA, can break confidentiality in order to safeguard other drivers (Option A). However, they must write to the patient before and after doing so (Option C). The doctor must act in the best interests of the community and therefore, if it is required, break confidentiality to safeguard the community as a whole; hence option D is the least appropriate answer.

21. **Correct Answer: A, B**

This is a tricky question. Your first natural response might be to respond in full, outlining the details of the case in order to correct the review (option C). However, this is inappropriate because you must not break patient confidentiality in such a way. Options A and B are the most appropriate first line options as they will both be able to give advice on how to proceed. Option D is not appropriate as other patients can read these comments and there is a risk that this might negatively impact on the reputation of your practice. Asking the practice manager to get the patient struck off the list would be a disproportionate and inappropriate step at this stage (option E).

22. **Correct Answer: A, B, D, C, E**

This is a very serious allegation and therefore to take the allegations no further is clearly the least appropriate option (option E). It would be prudent to discuss this situation immediately with your clinical supervisor (option A) or your defence union (option B). This incident will need reporting to the GMC (option D), but options A and B should occur first. Doctors should call the police (option C) should they believe a sexual assault has taken place. In this case more information is needed at this point and therefore this is ranked fourth.

23. **Correct Answer: A, B**

This is a tricky situation. On the one hand you do not want to jeopardise your relationship with the patient by being rude. However, you need to let the patient know that this is not an appropriate arena for discussing her medical issues. The other facet of this scenario is maintaining confidentiality which may be difficult if you discuss the case openly with the patient with other shoppers nearby. With this in mind options A and B are the most appropriate.

24. **Correct Answer: A, E, D, B, C**

If you make an error you should acknowledge it and apologize for it as soon as you can (option A). This error will likely delay the result of the investigation and therefore it would be prudent to inform your consultant (option E). Option D is an excellent measure to ensure that this incident isn't repeated, although it doesn't help solve the acute issue. Retaking the bloods in two weeks' time defeats the point of the follow up appointment (option B) and option C is clearly the least appropriate.

25. **Correct Answer: B, A, D, E, C**

An important part of the ST1 personal specification is the ability to manage time and tasks effectively. Therefore, the ability to prioritise clinical tasks is crucial if you are to do well in this exam. Here the pulseless patient (who is in cardiac arrest until proven otherwise) must be your top priority (option B). In reality there will be other staff around to help you and therefore the post-operative patient in option A (who you should have ranked second) could be attended to by another member of staff. However, for the purpose of these questions you do not have the luxury of discussing this. The phone call from biochemistry (option D) should be next as it could relate to a particularly worrying blood test result. As the patient in option E has their transport already there, this should be next. This leaves option C last which is understandable as it is of low clinical concern, and the question clearly states that you spoke to the relative at length yesterday.

26. **Correct Answer: C, E, B, A, D**

The ST1 personal specification states that two important qualities of a specialist trainee are the ability to manage time and prioritise. In this task you should deal with the clinically important tasks first, hence you should prioritise option C and then option E. The patient in option C may be having a heart attack and therefore you should attend the patient immediately as this is a medical emergency. The patient in option E needs to be attended to next as this patient sounds as though they are deteriorating and therefore prompt assessment is prudent. They may require a home visit or even emergency admission to hospital. After this, you should tackle tasks which are important and likely to distract you next. Therefore phoning your partner back should be your next consideration as this is likely to distract you from the other tasks you have remaining and additionally it is a task that may not take too long (option B). You should dictate your letters next as these are clinically important and any significant delay may impact negatively on patient care. Finally, option D should be addressed. Audit is an important part of quality improvement; however it is the least important in this scenario due to the more pressing clinical issues.

27. **Correct Answer: B, D, G**

This is a tricky situation. You will naturally want to help your friend but equally you cannot be seen to show them any favouritism. Ideally, as the patient is one of your best friends, you should ask someone else to see and treat them. Additionally, you have to maintain confidentiality about their case. Hence, options B, D and G are the most appropriate.

28. **Correct Answer: A, B, D, E, C**

By asking the current FY2 which presentations you can expect to see on a frequent basis (option A) you can guide your private study (option B). Option D is worthwhile as your consultant may be able to offer sage advice. Option E is a useful step but it doesn't tackle the acute issue of your impending on-call shift and therefore is ranked fourth. Option C is clearly the least appropriate option and therefore is ranked last.

29. **Correct Answer: A and B**

Prior to examining the patients you must gain consent to carry out the intimate examination which should be at least verbal and, ideally, written consent (options A and B). All of the other options are inappropriate.

30. **Correct Answer: C and D**

This question aims to test your knowledge of confidentiality. Your duty to the patient extends beyond death and therefore you must maintain confidentiality (option C). It would be sensible to inform your consultant of this media intrusion (option D). All of the other options would breach confidentiality and therefore are inappropriate.

31. Correct Answer: D, C, E, B, A

You should begin by exploring why the patient feels that this treatment would be of benefit (option D) and then explain that the patient has the right to a second opinion (option C). It would however be wise to involve your supervising GP at this point (option E). Option B is one of the least appropriate answers as you do not feel that the treatment is warranted, however it would allow further discussions with a specialist. Option A is the least appropriate answer.

32. Correct Answer: A , E

You should avoid prescribing to family or people you know well unless it is unavoidable. Here the best options would be to involve the GP or the palliative care team who would be best suited to help (options A and E). To call an ambulance or arrange a hospital admission would be against her wishes to stay at home.

33. Correct Answer: C, B, A, D, E

It is unlikely that as an FY2 doctor you will have the clinical experience to confidently treat a gunshot wound. Hence option C is the most appropriate closely followed by option B. The GMC states that you should inform the police of any gun or knife wound seen in hospital. Usually, you shouldn't give the patient's details (option A). Option D and E are the least appropriate options, in that order as the first would require you to divulge the patient's details and the second would go against the GMC's guidance on this type of injury.

34. Correct Answer: D, A, C, E, B

This is a difficult situation. The task here is to act empathetically and sympathetically within the law. You should start by exploring his reasons for his request (option D) and then discuss whether there are any symptoms that you could relieve or treat (option A). It would be reasonable to suggest that a Counsellor or Psychologist might be able to help him come to terms with what has happened (option C) but is also important to explain to him that it would be illegal for you to help him die (option E). It is also illegal to encourage assisted suicide and therefore option B must be ranked last.

35. Correct Answer: A, F

It is important not to damage your relationship with the nurse in this situation and therefore option C is not a correct answer. Equally it would be inappropriate for you to examine her or order any investigations in your role as her colleague. In this scenario you should explain why you cannot do this (option F), and suggest she sees her GP (option A) as they will be best placed to investigate further. Because of the chronicity of the problem, acute presentation to A&E would not be appropriate (option B).

36. **Correct Answer: B, C**

It is important to respect patients' autonomy. However, in this situation you should ensure that the patient has all of the facts available to her to ensure she is in a position to reach a fully informed decision (option B). It would be a good idea to explore alternative treatments too at this stage (option C).

37. **Correct Answer: A, D**

Being a junior doctor can be a stressful and at times traumatic experience. When you are struggling it is important to be able to have a plan in order to cope. The GMC guidance mandates that a doctor must manage their own health so as to be able to effectively treat their patients. The most appropriate answers here therefore are A and D.

38. **Correct Answer: C, D, B, E, A**

It is crucial in this situation to remain calm and polite throughout the encounter (option C). It would be worthwhile to explore exactly why the patient is demanding the drug and to collect some background information (option D). By this stage it may well be necessary to involve your supervisor to help you manage this difficult patient (option B). Refusing to treat the patient at all may inflame the situation further (option E). However, you should not prescribe any drug just because a patient demands it and therefore option A is the least appropriate option.

39. **Correct Answer: A, C, E**

It is important here to show the nurse that you have taken what she has said on board (option E) and then act on it appropriately (option A). It would be very reasonable to ask your registrar for advice (option C). To tell the nurse that she should speak to the FY1 herself may damage your relationship with the nursing staff, and equally to speak to the FY1 publicly may damage your relationship with him. Option F may need to be undertaken eventually. However, it would seem to be a disproportionate action given this one isolated incident. As an FY2 you have a leadership role within the team and therefore Option G is inappropriate.

40. **Correct Answer: B, D, A, C, E**

You are obliged to pull over to help but you should ensure your own safety when doing so (option B). Calling an ambulance early is crucial so that it can be *en route* while you assess the patient (option D). You should then treat the cyclist (option A). Contacting your defence union (option C) may or may not be something you wish to do but either way you should not let this delay treating the patient in the first instance. Finally, option E in this situation would be unacceptable.

41. Correct Answer: A, E

Exposing patient details in this way, however accidental, is a serious matter. In this situation you should dispose of the list confidentially (option E) in the first instance. Secondly, you should let the hospital's clinical governance lead know (option A) about the incident so that measures to minimise the risk of this occurring again can be put in place. Neither options B or C are appropriate for reasons of confidentiality and option D is not appropriate as you need to ensure this doesn't happen again.

42. Correct Answer: A, D, C, B, E

This question allows an opportunity to demonstrate several characteristics which are mentioned on the personal specification (problem solving and conceptual thinking for example). The first thing you should do here is to call the police (option A) as they will then try to find the car and hopefully prevent the drugs or patient notes falling into the wrong hands. Calling your supervisor at this point is wise as you will need help in managing the situation (option D). You should inform the patient as soon as possible that their notes are in the stolen car (option C), before arranging a replacement vehicle (option B). Finally, you must complete an incident form about this case (option E).

43. Correct Answer: D, A, C, E, B

This question is about showing your capacity to update your knowledge – which is a crucial aspect of the ST1 personal specification. An e-learning module (option D) is likely to be well structured and allow you to gain a certificate for your e-portfolio. This makes it preferential to "reading around" the subject (option A). It would be wise to do these steps prior to asking your registrar to help (option C). You will undoubtedly improve your knowledge over the coming months, but it is not enough just to rely on ad hoc learning (option E). To do nothing is clearly the worst answer (option B).

44. Correct Answer: B, D

This question tests your ability to work effectively within a team. The nurse practitioner in this scenario is essentially bullying you and this needs to be dealt with appropriately. Although it may be challenging, the most appropriate first line option is to speak to the nurse practitioner directly (option D). Following this, you should involve your clinical supervisor for his/her advice (option B).

45. Correct Answer: B, E, C, A, D

Patients have the right to autonomy and this extends to opting against treatment. Your role in this situation is to ensure that the patient is fully informed of the consequences of his decision (option B) and to answer any questions he may have (option E). Ultimately, however, you should respect the patient's decision (option C). Adults are assumed to have capacity until proven otherwise and there is nothing in this question to suggest that he lacks capacity. It would be wise to inform his GP of this decision (option A). It would be entirely inappropriate to treat the patient against his will and therefore option D is ranked last.

46. **Correct Answer: E, B, D, C, A**

You should start in this case by discussing the patient's reasons for being stressed (option E) as you may be able to treat him more successfully by knowing the precipitating factor. During a discussion of how it is affecting him he may admit to the assault that took place last week (option B). It is important to find out if there are any children at home because there may also be underlying child protection issues (option D). Having gathered all of this information you should discuss it with your supervisor as this situation is potentially volatile and may require the input of an experienced clinician (option C). By divulging his wife's allegations to the patient you are both breaking confidentiality and potentially putting her at risk. Therefore option A is ranked last.

47. **Correct Answer: E, A, C, D, B**

As a doctor you are expected to protect patient dignity and ensure patient safety. This scenario tackles both of these issues. You should raise the issue of hand washing (option E) immediately as it is essentially a patient safety issue. Option A is a very straightforward measure which you can easily perform to ensure patient dignity is maintained. Discussing the situation with your consultant (option C) would be appropriate, as the registrar is effectively acting on your consultant's behalf. Raising the issue with the GMC would be quite disproportionate at this stage and therefore Option D is ranked fourth. However, Option B is the least appropriate answer as it fails to tackle the issues regarding patient dignity and safety.

48. **Correct Answer: B, E**

All doctors are required to mentor junior colleagues and this extends to medical students too. Here you should agree to mentor the student (option B) and try to establish their learning objectives (option E) as this will enable you to establish which tasks will be most appropriate for the student to help with. You will have to explain to the student that you have a busy day ahead and therefore you may not be able to teach them as much as you would like to.

49. **Correct Answer: C, A, D, E, B**

Here the key is the maxim – "first do no harm." Clearly you do not know how to prescribe this drug and therefore you have a plethora of options before you. A good starting point would be the hospital's protocol for the drug (option C). Failing this the BNF is an excellent next option as it shows you are willing to learn and have initiative (option A). At this point, if you are still struggling, it would now be reasonable to consult your registrar for help (option D). Options E and B are last. The order here was decided on the fact that it is likely better not to prescribe the drug erroneously than to attempt to prescribe it without help and potentially cause the patient harm.

50.   **Correct Answer: B, A, D, E, C**

The most important objective in this scenario is to ensure that the care of the patient in question does not suffer as a result of this error and there-fore option B is the most appropriate. You should then give your colleague an opportunity to explain why she had not handed the patient over (option A). There may be a good reason why this error occurred and therefore it is important to resolve this. Talking the case through with your consultant would be worthwhile (option D) and the completion of an incident form (option E) may help to raise the issue of handover and help prevent such an occurrence happening again.

51.   **Correct Answer: B, D**

The most important thing to do in this situation is to commence CPR (option B). You should call the crash team as soon as possible (option D), and it would make sense to request that one of the bystanders does this while you contin-ue your resuscitation efforts. Note the wording of the question "which would be the first **two** things you would do" – you may do more than two in reality, but the correct answer here is what you would do initially.

52.   **Correct Answer: B, D, C, A, E**

Here you should maintain a good working relationship with the ward clerk by acknowledging her concerns and addressing them accordingly (option B). It is a great opportunity to show your ability to delegate (option D). Option C is worthwhile but doesn't offer an immediate solution to the outstanding issue. Both options A and E are poor answers but to inaccurately complete the discharge summaries is the worst option here. Discharge summaries are crucial for continuity of care and clinical decisions are made on their content and therefore option E is ranked last.

53.   **Correct Answer: A, D**

The "sick note" has in fact been rebranded the "fit note", although many patients will still refer to it in old terms. The most appropriate measure in this scenario is to explain to the patient that he can self-certificate for up to 7 days (option D). It would also be wise to give him advice about the manage-ment of his illness (option A). It would be inappropriate at this stage to issue him with a "fit note."

54.   **Correct Order: D, B, C, A, E**

This is a difficult situation. You should confirm initially that the patient has indeed died (option D) and then contact your supervisor for advice (option B). You should then inform the coroner via the police (option C then A).

This is particularly important as the patient has not been seen recently by a doctor. You should also then inform the next of kin (option E).

55.   **Correct Answer: A, B, E, C, D**

It can be really useful to take photographs of interesting or useful cases for educational purposes. You should start by explaining why you would like to take these photos (option A) and then, ideally, gain written consent (option B). If you are unable to gain written consent for some reason then oral consent may suffice (option E) although it is less preferable. Most hospitals now have a medical photography department (option C) who will take the images for you. The least appropriate answer here is to take the images yourself on your phone (option D).

Clinical Problem Solving answers and explanations

1. **Correct Answer: B. Anterior uveitis**
   Anterior uveitis is a common cause of "red eye". This painful condition affects visual acuity and is associated with seronegative spondyloarthropathies such as ankylosing spondylitis. A hypopyon is a collection of inflammatory cells seen in the anterior chamber of the eye and is often present in anterior uveitis – this is best seen using a slit lamp.

2. **Correct Answer: D. Bitemporal hemianopia**
   This patient is displaying symptoms which could be consistent with a pituitary prolactinoma. Symptoms include those secondary to the secretion of prolactin (lethargy, weight gain and galactorrhoea) and, later, local pressure effects of the tumour itself (headache, visual field defects). Because of the position of the pituitary gland the part of the optic tract most vulnerable to pressure from a tumour is the optic chiasm. Hence, a bitemporal hemianopia is the most likely visual field defect of the available options.

3. **Correct Answer: B. Pertussis**
   Live vaccines should not be given to pregnant women and therefore rubella, measles, mumps and BCG should not be given. Pertussis can be given to pregnant mums and is an excellent way of helping to protect the baby from whooping cough.

4. **Correct Answer: A. Human Parainfluenza Virus**
   Cervical cancer is associated with human papillomavirus (HPV) and not human parainfluenza virus infection. More specifically, associations exist with several HPV strains including 16, 18. All of the other options are recognised risk factors for the development of cervical cancer.

5. **Correct Answer: A. 500 mcg of 1:1000 adrenaline I.M**
   Initial treatment for anaphylaxis is 500 mcg of 1:1000 adrenaline intramuscularly (I.M.). Intravenous adrenaline can be used in anaphylaxis treatment but the UK Resuscitation Council guidelines state that that this should only be done by a specialist.

6. **Correct Answer: E. Altered conscious level**
   All of the options for this question are indicators of a severe asthma attack but only option E would indicate a life-threatening attack. The BTS guidelines give clear, objective assessments for what constitutes a life-threatening asthma attack. These include, but are not limited to, altered conscious level, exhaustion, arrhythmia, hypotension, PEF <33% and a silent chest.

7. **Correct Answer: B. Amlodipine**
   According to NICE guidelines for hypertension management, in patients who are over 55-years-old or who are of African or Caribbean origin, the

first choice management is a calcium channel blocker (unless contraindicated). Hence, Amlodipine is the correct answer.

8. **Correct Answer: G. Ramipril**

Angioedema is a recognised side-effect of ACE-inhibitors.

9. **Correct Answer: E. Amlodipine**

Calcium channel blockers, such as Amlodipine, can cause peripheral oedema.

10. **Correct Answer: C. Propanolol**

Beta-blockers can cause cold extremities. This unwanted side effect is more likely with a non-selective beta-blocker like propranolol.

11. **Correct Answer: D. Clarithromycin and Simvastatin**

Recent studies have shown that concomitant use of clarithromycin with simvastatin can increase the risk of the development of rhabdomyolysis.

12. **Correct Answer: G. Pancreatitis**

Pancreatitis is a recognised complication of ERCP.

13. **Correct Answer: D Biliary colic**

Strictly speaking, biliary colic is a symptom rather than a disease. It is the term given to symptomatic gall stones which typically presents with spasmodic pain in the right upper quadrant of the abdomen.

14. **Correct Answer: F. Cholelithiasis**

Cholelithiasis refers to the formation of gallstones within the gall bladder.

15. **Correct Answer: A. Koilonychia**

This patient is clearly anaemic as evidenced by both her clinical examination and the history of heavy menstrual loss. Koilonychia are spoon-shaped nails which are associated with iron-deficiency anaemia.

16. **Correct Answer: D. Emollients**

Emollients are the mainstay of eczema treatment and would be the first choice for this patient. Following this, mild topical steroids would be a reasonable addition. The other options in this list are reserved for moderate and severe eczema.

17. **Correct Answer: E. Benign Paroxysmal Positional Vertigo (BPPV)**

Benign Paroxysmal Positional Vertigo (BPPV) is a condition which causes sudden severe attacks of vertigo. The Dix-Hallpike test can be used in its diagnosis. Treatment options vary widely from the well-known Epley manoeuvres, through to medication and (in very rare cases) even surgery.

18. **Correct Answer: D. Central retinal artery occlusion**

Central retinal artery occlusion is an important cause of visual loss. Thrombus is often the cause (although not the only cause) and therefore it is more likely in patients who have risk factors for thrombus formation e.g. atrial fibrillation. The classic retinal signs seen are diffuse hypopigmentation with a well-defined area of hyperpigmentation in the macula; commonly referred to as a "red dot".

19. **Correct Answer: A. No further investigation required**
This patient has symptoms of hyperglycaemia therefore it is diagnostic if his venous glucose level is found to be elevated only once (fasting ≥7mmol/l or random ≥11 mmol/l). Had he not been symptomatic then another test (from the options in the question) on a different day would be required to confirm the diagnosis. HbA1c can be used in this instance but there are certain patient groups (e.g. children) where it cannot be used.

20. **Correct Answer: C. Hyperkalaemia**
Addison's disease has a strong association with other autoimmune diseases and is more common in females. It is caused by primary adrenocortical insufficiency.

21. **Correct Answer: G. Spermatocele**
Spermatoceles are benign lesions which usually arise from the epididymis. They transilluminate as they are fluid filled. Hydroceles also transilluminate but are usually anterior to the testicle.

22. **Correct Answer: D. Testicular tumour**
This patient has a testicular tumour until proven otherwise. The large craggy mass, along with the patient's symptomatic back pain (which could be due to metastasis), should prompt urgent further investigation and referral.

23. **Correct Answer: F. Testicular torsion**
The twisting, and associated ischaemia, of a testis is acutely painful, however, due to their embryological origin this pain can often be felt in the abdomen. Therefore it is crucial to examine the external genitalia of boys presenting with abdominal pain.

24. **Correct Answer: E. Sitagliptin**
The group of medications which are DPP-4 inhibitors are colloquially known as "gliptins." Their use is associated with an increased risk of acute pancreatitis; therefore patients should be warned about this when commencing the drug.

25. **Correct Answer: C. Pulmonary embolus**
All of the above conditions can cause shortness of breath, tachycardia and hypoxia, so all are possibilities. However, the question asks for the most likely cause of the patient's symptoms. Pulmonary embolism is the most likely as the patient has a concomitant malignancy, the shortness of breath was of sudden onset, and he is tachycardic, hypoxic, tachypnoeic and has no other past medical history. There is no mention of any infective feature which makes pneumonia less likely. The likelihood of congestive cardiac

failure and myocardial infarction are reduced by the lack of past medical history and there are no particular risk factors for pneumothorax.

26. **Correct Answer: E. Appendicitis**
In this scenario the clinical examination is crucial in deciding the correct answer. Appendicitis can be difficult to diagnose in children, and therefore it should always be considered as a differential in patients who present with abdominal pain.

27. **Correct Answer: D. Edwards' syndrome**
Caused by trisomy 18, children with Edwards' syndrome have the characteristic features described in the question. The prominent heels are often referred to as "Rocker bottom feet."

28. **Correct Answer: E. Turner's syndrome**
Patients with Turner's syndrome are female and are missing a sex chromosome (45X). They often have associated cardiac abnormalities.

29. **Correct Answer: G. Down syndrome**
Down syndrome is caused by trisomy 21. It is commonly screened for during the ante-natal period.

30. **Correct Answer: F. Naloxone**
Naloxone has long been recognised as a potent antagonist to opiates.

31. **Correct Answer: B. Flumazenil**
Flumazenil is a GABA receptor antagonist and as such it can be used in the management of benzodiazepine overdose.

32. **Correct Answer: C. N-acetylcysteine**
Of the available options in this question N-acetylcysteine is the correct answer as it is sometimes (though not always) used in the management of paracetamol overdose.

33. **Correct Answer: C. Combined oral contraceptive pill (COCP)**
All of the options in this question are recognised risk factors for the development of endometrial cancer apart from use of the combined oral contraceptive pill (COCP), which has been linked to a reduction in risk.

34. **Correct Answer: A. Progesterone only pill (POP)**
The Mirena intrauterine system (IUS) may be difficult to fit due to her past medical history of fibroids. The combined oral contraceptive pill is contraindicated as she is over 35 years old and smokes ›15 cigarettes per day (as per the UK MEC Guidelines). Both Implanon and Depo-Provera would be difficult in this patient due to her needle phobia. This leaves the progesterone only pill as the most suitable contraception for this patient.

35. Correct answer: A. Oily skin

Isotretinoin is a retinoid used in the management of acne. Recognised side effects include all of the options given in the question apart from oily skin. On the contrary, retinoids cause markedly dry skin. Of particular importance in female patients is the high risk of teratogenicity and therefore patients must be carefully counselled with regards to contraception.

36. Correct Answer: E. Oesophageal cancer

The most likely answer is Oesophageal cancer. Iranians have a much higher incidence of this cancer and the progressive nature of the dysphagia accompanied by weight loss and anaemia is highly suggestive of the diagnosis. Additionally, the patient in this scenario has been exposed to high levels of alcohol and smoke during his lifetime, both of which increase his risk of developing oesophageal cancer. Chagas' disease (American Trypanosomiasis) is a parasitic infection common in South American populations. It is therefore unlikely in this case unless there is a compatible travel history. Stroke would be unlikely to cause progressive dysphagia, and achalasia would not be consistent with the patient's anaemia or substantial weight loss. The same is true for a thoracic aortic aneurysm.

37. Correct Answer: D. Bladder cancer

This patient has been exposed to two major risk factors for the development of bladder cancer; smoking and chemicals used in the textiles industry. This history combined with his presenting complaint of macroscopic haematuria and weight loss must make bladder cancer high on your list of differential diagnoses.

38. Correct Answer: G. Pre-eclampsia

Pre-eclampsia is much more common in primigravida women. This patient requires immediate admission under the obstetric team.

39. Correct Answer A. Orthostatic proteinuria

Patients with orthostatic proteinuria have measurable urinary protein on standing which resolves when supine. Hence the negative protein tests in the morning, and positive tests later in the day. It is a benign condition which typically affects children and adolescents.

40. Correct Answer: B. 10

This patient's score is 10, based on Eyes = 1, Verbal = 3, Motor = 6

41. Correct Answer: A. Type I hypersensitivity

Type I hypersensitivity refers to IgE-mediated reactions such as allergic rhinoconjunctivitis and anaphylaxis.

42. **Correct Answer: D. 3rd degree haemorrhoids**

Haemorrhoids which require manual reduction are classified as 3rd degree. This patient has risk factors for the development of prolapsed haemorrhoids (COPD and previous vaginal deliveries).

43. **Correct Answer: E. Borderline personality disorder**

Personality disorders are difficult to diagnose as there is often overlap in the symptoms between classifications. In this case however, the patient has many of the hallmarks of a borderline personality disorder including impulsive behaviour, self-harm, intense (but short lived) relationships, and occasional auditory hallucinations.

44. **Correct Answer: A. Diclofenac**

Gout is excruciating, so the first goal of management should focus on symptom relief. NICE recommend NSAIDs in the first instance. Allopurinol should not be started in the acute phase because it may precipitate further attacks. Instead allopurinol should be used to prevent recurrence, but only after the initial attack has settled. Colchicine should be used if NSAIDs are contraindicated or not tolerated.

45. **Correct Answer: D. Three**

The ABCD2 score is used to aid management of patients with TIA by estimating the patient's risk of having a subsequent stroke. This patient scores a point for age, blood pressure and speech disturbance and therefore his score is three which would put him in the low risk category.

46. **Correct Answer: C. Cluster headache**

This headache is more common in male smokers and is usually unilateral and associated with other symptoms such as eye watering or nasal blockage.

47. **Correct Answer: A. Tension headache**

Tension headaches are more common in female patients and are often worse in the evenings. Patients often describe the pain as being like "a tight band."

48. **Correct Answer: B. Migraine**

Migraines can take many forms. The patient in this question is describing a classical migraine with aura. Migraines are typically unilateral and can occur with or without visual aura (zig-zag lines across the vision of the patient in this case).

49. **Correct Answer: B. 25%**

Cystic fibrosis is an autosomal recessive condition and therefore the offspring of parents who are both carriers (not sufferers) have a one in four (25%) chance that their child will develop the disease.

50. Correct Answer: A. 0%

Haemophilia A is an X-linked recessive disease and therefore cannot be passed from father to son as the father provides the unaffected 'Y Chromosome' and the mother provides the 'X chromosome'.

51. Correct Answer: C. PHQ-9

The PHQ-9 is a patient questionnaire used in primary care to assess depression. AUDIT (Alcohol Use Disorders Identification Test) is used in the assessment of alcohol use and PDI is the "Psoriasis Disability Index". QCPC is the "Questionnaire of Chronic illness in Primary Care" and the PSQ is a "Patient Satisfaction Questionnaire" which can be used as part of the appraisal process for GPs.

52. Correct Answer: A. Acute onset over hours

Dementia and delirium can be difficult to differentiate, and often overlap. However, the history in delirium is often much more acute when compared to dementia which, usually, takes weeks, months or even years to develop. Dementia is irreversible and progressive and patients usually have normal attention. Delirium by contrast often fluctuates and patients can recover well.

53. Correct Answer: E. Admit the patient acutely under the neurosurgical team

This patient has cauda equina syndrome until proven otherwise. This would likely be due to bony metastases to the spine from his prostate cancer. He needs immediate neurosurgical assessment and imaging and therefore should be acutely admitted under this team as an emergency.

54. Correct Answer: D. Median nerve

This patient has carpal tunnel syndrome which is caused by compression of the median nerve. Symptoms are typically worse at night. This particular patient has two recognised risk factors for the development of the condition: diabetes and pregnancy. Tinel's test is positive when reproduction of the symptoms is brought about by lightly tapping over the nerve at the palmar aspect of the wrist.

55. Correct Answer: A. Radial nerve

Because the course of the radial nerve is in such close proximity to the humeral shaft it is particularly vulnerable to fractures here. Injuries cause a classic "wrist drop" and numbness in the distribution of the nerve.

56. Correct Answer: E. Axillary nerve

The axillary nerve is vulnerable to damage when shoulder dislocations occur. The area of numbness described in the question is typical of an axillary nerve injury and is often referred to as the "regimental badge area."

57. **Correct Answer: D. Trigger finger**

Trigger finger is caused by a nodule on the tendon sheath which prevents extension by jamming the finger in the flexed position. If it is troublesome it may require surgical management.

58. **Correct Answer: B. Dressler's syndrome**

Dressler's syndrome is a recognised complication of myocardial infarction which typically occurs approximately two weeks after the initial event. It is caused by autoantibodies to the myocardium. It is usually self-limiting but it frequently requires a period of inpatient observation.

59. **Correct Answer: C. Indirect inguinal hernia**

Indirect inguinal hernias are more common than direct hernias. They traverse the inguinal canal and therefore, after reduction, can typically be controlled by pressure over the internal inguinal ring.

60. **Correct Answer: E. Paraumbilical hernia**

These hernias are much more common in female patients. They are prone to strangulation and incarceration and therefore often require pre-emptive surgical repair.

61. **Correct Answer: D. Parastomal hernia**

Hernias which develop around the site of stomas are referred to as parastomal hernias. They are a recognised complication of stoma formation. In most cases they are symptomless and conservative management can be used. However, in some cases surgical intervention is the treatment of choice. The patient in this question is more at risk of parastomal hernias as he is obese.

62. **Correct Answer: D. Gilbert's syndrome**

Gilbert's syndrome is a common benign condition which causes hyperbilirubinemia. The condition is often exacerbated by concurrent infection (as in the patient in the question) or may be noted on routine blood tests.

63. **Correct Answer: A. Pinguecula**

A pinguecula is a benign lesion which is often caused by exposure to UV light. Under normal circumstances they require no active treatment. A pinguecula does not encroach over the cornea which helps to differentiate it from a pterygium.

64. **Correct Answer: D. Presence of immunosuppression**

The Centor criteria are a useful way for a general practitioner to objectively assess the likelihood of tonsillitis being caused by streptococcus. This is important as most cases of tonsillitis are viral and therefore use of these criteria can help to avoid unnecessary antibiotic prescribing. Additionally, it helps to highlight those patients who would most benefit from antibiotics and may be at higher risk of post-streptococcal sequelae. Immunosuppression is not taken into account.

65. **Correct Answer: A. I.M. Benzylpenicillin**

This is a medical emergency. In cases of suspected meningococcal meningitis, I.M. Benzylpenicillin should be administered pre-hospital as there is evidence to show that this improves morbidity and mortality.

66. **Correct Answer: D. Insert a cannula into the mid clavicular line, second intercostal space on the right side.**

This patient has developed a tension pneumothorax which requires immediate decompression using a wide bore cannula. This patient's chest is hyperresonant, with reduced breath sounds on the right and the trachea is deviated away from this side therefore it is the right side that needs decompressing. This patient will eventually need a chest drain, but acutely they require urgent decompression. To order a chest X-ray or to continue your assessment would only delay lifesaving treatment further.

67. **Correct Answer: E. A 60 year old patient with no major medical problems**

The National Institute for Health and Care Excellence (NICE) recommend the seasonal influenza vaccination be offered to certain vulnerable groups. All of the groups in the scenario should be offered the vaccination apart from the healthy 60 year old, as routine vaccination is only offered from the age of 65. All pregnant women, regardless of gestation, should be offered the vaccination.

68. **Answer: D. Sulfasalazine**

Disease-modifying anti-rheumatic drugs (DMARDs) have been a revelation in the management of a wide range of rheumatological conditions. However, they are not without their flaws as they have many side effects. Sulfasalazine has been shown to produce oligospermia in some male patients. Fortunately it is usually reversible on stopping the drug.

69. **Answer: D. Malar flush**

Malar flush is associated with mitral stenosis and not aortic regurgitation. Aortic regurgitation (AR) has many causes including congenital, infectious and autoimmune and therefore can present as a chronic or acute problem depending on the aetiology. There are many physical signs which can be present with AR. Collapsing pulse (also known as "water hammer pulse"), prominent carotid pulsation, Quincke's sign (nail bed pulsation) and wide pulse pressure are all associated with AR.

70. **Correct Answer: G. Cranial Nerve VII (The facial nerve)**

The patient in this scenario is suffering from a Bell's palsy. This poorly understood condition leads to paralysis of the facial nerve (cranial nerve VII). It is a lower motor neurone problem and therefore the patient cannot raise the eyebrow on the affected side.

71. Correct Answer: F. Cranial nerve VI (The abducens nerve)

The patient in this scenario has developed a mononeuropathy second-ary to his poorly controlled diabetes. On this occasion it is the abducens nerve (cranial nerve VI) that is affected. This nerve supplies the lateral rectus muscle and therefore explains the inability to abduct the affected eye.

72. Correct Answer: E. Cranial nerve V (The trigeminal nerve)

This patient is describing the typical history of trigeminal neuralgia which involves the trigeminal nerve (cranial nerve V). It is a chronic condition which is characterised by severe bouts of pain which are often precipitated by seemingly innocuous stimuli.

73. Correct Answer: E. Osteoporosis

The risk of all of the options given in this question are potentially increased by HRT apart from osteoporosis, the risk of which is reduced.

74. Correct Answer: D. Metronidazole

Many cases of bacterial vaginosis (BV) spontaneously resolve. However, the treatment of choice is Metronidazole. Regular vaginal douching is not recommended as it can severely upset the normal vaginal flora and can cause or worsen BV.

75. Correct Answer: E. Syphilis

All of the options are notifiable diseases apart from syphilis. A full list can be found on the HPA website (*Appendix*).

76. Correct Answer: D. Placental abruption

This patient is showing several features of placental abruption. She has experienced sudden onset, constant abdominal pain with associated mater-nal shock. In conjunction with the physical examination (hard uterus) and inability to locate foetal heartbeat an obstetric emergency should be declared and an urgent specialist assessment is required. Placental abruption can be concealed (as in this case) or revealed (in which case there would be the passage of blood from the vagina).

77. Correct Answer: A. *Escherichia coli*

This patient is suffering from a urinary tract infection. The most common organism therefore is *Escherichia coli*.

78. Correct Answer: C. *Streptococcus viridans*

Streptococcus viridans is a recognised cause of bacterial endocarditis.

79. Correct Answer: F. *Pseudomonas aeruginosa*

Pseudomonas aeruginosa and *staphylococcus aureus* are the most common causative organisms in otitis externa.

80. **Correct Answer: A. Long acting beta agonist (LABA)**
This is a slightly tricky question as you do not have a huge amount of information about his symptoms or current dosage. However, this is deliberate as the question aims to test your knowledge of the British Thoracic Society (BTS) asthma guidelines. These state that the next step should be the addition of a LABA and, depending on the response to this, only then consider increasing the dose of the inhaled steroid. The other treatments come much later in the treatment ladder.

81. **Correct Answer: B. Stress incontinence**
This patient is describing typical symptoms of stress incontinence. Her obstetric history may have predisposed her to this. Management initially centres on floor exercises but may eventually require surgical intervention.

82. **Correct Answer: B. Carotid body tumour**
These tumours, although rare, are important to diagnose because of their potential for local invasion and eventual metastasis.

83. **Correct Answer: H. Branchial cyst**
These typically occur in young adults and require surgical management.

84. **Correct Answer: F. Goitre**
This patient is showing signs of Graves' disease and therefore the most likely answer is goitre.

85. **Correct Answer: E. Intussusception**
Intussusception is more common in boys than girls. Initial management is with resuscitation and then either medical or surgical approaches according to the clinical condition of the child.

86. **Correct Answer: A. Dermovate**
Dermovate is classed as a very potent topical steroid. In ascending order of potency the creams mentioned in this question would be: mild – Hydrocortisone 1%; moderate – Eumovate; potent – Betnovate and Elocon; and very potent – Dermovate.

87. **Correct Answer: C. Minimum of 6 months**
According to the DVLA guidelines, following a first unprovoked seizure, a patient with a group one licence (i.e. car/motorcycle) must not drive for 6 months following the date of the seizure. This could be increased to 12 months depending on the results of investigations.

88. **Correct Answer: D. No more than 21 units of alcohol per week**
The Department of Health guidelines suggest that men should not exceed 21 units of alcohol per week (and no more than 4 units in any one day), and that women should not exceed 14 units of alcohol per week (and no more than 3

units in any one day). They also recommend 2 alcohol-free days per week for both men and women.

89. **Correct Answer: D. Simmonds' test**
During Simmonds' test the clinician (with the patient kneeling on a chair or lying flat on their front) squeezes the affected calf. If this does not cause plantar flexion of the foot then this is said to be a positive test and supports the diagnosis of a ruptured Achilles tendon.

90. **Correct Answer: D. Haemoglobin concentration**
The haemoglobin measurement is decreased in normal pregnancy due to dilution.

91. **Correct Answer: A. Tetracycline**
Tetracycline should not be prescribed to children under 12 years old due to the risk of dental staining and (rarely) dental hypoplasia. It also should not be given to pregnant or breast-feeding women.

92. **Correct Answer: B. Phimosis**
This common condition can resolve spontaneously, however surgical intervention (in the form of circumcision) is sometimes required, particularly if infections are a problem.

93. **Correct Answer: B. Ankylosing spondylitis (AS)**
This patient is exhibiting the typical history of AS in which a young man presents with low back pain which is worse in the morning and improves with stretching/exercise. AS is initially investigated with plain X-ray and blood tests; early involvement of a rheumatologist and physiotherapist can be helpful. Other features of the disease can include (but are not limited to) ocular symptoms such as iritis or uveitis, and cardiovascular involvement such as with aortic regurgitation.

94. **Correct Answer: D. Cyclosporin**
A recognised side effect of Cyclosporin is hypertrichosis (excessive hair growth). Incidentally, Azathioprine, Mycophenolate mofetil and Gold can all cause hair loss.

95. **Correct Answer: E. Seborrhoeic keratosis**
The most likely diagnosis here is seborrhoeic keratosis. These are benign lesions which can occur anywhere on the skin. They typically have a "stuck on" appearance. Often it is enough to reassure patients that they are innocent lesions, however if they are troublesome they can be removed easily.

96. **Correct Answer: A. Saphena varix**
A saphena varix is a dilatation of the long saphenous vein at the point of insertion to the femoral vein.

97. Correct Answer: C. VIII

Warfarin acts as a vitamin K antagonist. Clotting factors II, VII, IX and X are all vitamin K-dependent clotting factors. Warfarin also acts on protein C, protein S and protein Z.

98. Correct Answer: A. Diabetic ketoacidosis

This patient has diabetic ketoacidosis (DKA) as it meets the triad of criteria required to diagnose it (hyperglycaemia, acidosis, and ketosis). This is a medical emergency. It is universally accepted that the most important first step in managing DKA is appropriate fluid resuscitation.

99. Correct Answer: C. Four Weeks

The DVLA recommend 4 weeks' abstention from driving following a myocardial infarction (M.I.), but the patient is not required to directly inform the DVLA of their M.I.

100. Correct Answer: C. Sarcoma

Paget's disease of the bone is a condition which typically affects the elderly and often leads to a raised alkaline phosphatase. These patients are at increased risk of developing sarcoma.

Stage 3 practice paper answers and discussions

Discussion of Clinical Scenario 1

This scenario is typical of the sort of scenario which you might face with the simulated patient. Ultimately there is no 'right answer' to this (or any other) scenario and therefore points below represent some ideas to consider:

- Remember it is not a clinical exam as such so resist the temptation to take a clinical history about abdominal pain. It will get you no credit. The scenario states that the patient has already been seen by a consultant and that your involvement regards her desire to self-discharge.

- It's really important to show your empathetic side in this scenario. Phrases like "I can see that you're really worried" or "I can understand why you're feeling anxious" show the patient, and crucially the examiner, that you are empathetic.

- Open questions early on should have unearthed why the patient was worried (i.e. about the prospect of surgery) and if you used the "Ideas, Concerns and Expectations model" (ICE) then you should have hopefully unearthed that the basis of the patient's fear was the recent loss of her grandfather following surgery.

- This would have offered you a great opportunity to show your ability to work around a problem and reassure the patient. For example, by explaining that the decision to undergo surgery hadn't even been made yet and that she is being admitted for further assessment could help. Offering reassurance that repair of an abdominal aortic aneurysm in an elderly man is a much more risky operation than an appendicectomy in a fit young patient would also be a good thing to explore.

- It would have been excellent to explore the patient's support network and by doing so you may then have learned that having her mum there to support her would be a great help in managing her anxiety. This could have allowed you to take responsibility of a task by offering to phone her mum for example.

- It would also have been reasonable to explain to the patient that you can't keep her in hospital against her wishes but that medical advice would be to stay.

- Summarise what you have talked about and allow the patient to ask any questions she might have.

- By agreeing on the plan going forward you should hopefully have reassured her about staying for the further assessments.

Discussion of Clinical Scenario 2

The co-worker scenario can be difficult as it is very possible that you have never faced this sort of situation in real life. This is in stark contrast to the scenarios which involve a patient or relative/carer which you are much more likely to have faced in your everyday practice. Here are some things to consider regarding this particular scenario:

- Don't be put off by instructions with very little information like this example. This can work to your advantage as you will not have any preconceived ideas of what to expect.

- There are many facets to this scenario but a logical approach will help. It can seem overwhelming to begin a consultation like this with minimal instruction and only ten minutes in which to grapple with the countless issues that you will no doubt need to consider. However, if you approach the problem logically you will be more equipped to deal with the scenario.

- As always, start with open questions and look for hidden clues or agenda. This will give you a good idea as to which direction the consultation should go.

- Remember to leave closed questions until later in the consultation.

- There are plenty of opportunities here to show empathy to this co-worker. Again, by reflecting her emotions back at her you can show the examiner your empathy. For example "I can see that you're upset by this" or "I can understand how hard this must be for you."

- It is important in this scenario to thoroughly explore the patient's support network. In this scenario the patient's husband and daughter are both impacted by her current problems at work and as such this needs addressing.

- You should ideally ask about sleep, drinking, smoking etc. and you would be quite justified in exploring Wendy's mood (including if appropriate a risk assessment).

- However, while it's important to talk about mood here try to resist turning it into a consultation.

- In this case Wendy's expectation is that you might be able to help her in managing her current situation. It's important that you establish this as part of your ICE approach.

- You can exhibit your ability to work around a problem in many ways here. Perhaps you could discuss ways in which to address the issue with her management (e.g. formally or through a union).

- Additionally, this scenario offers an excellent opportunity to arrange follow up. Having agreed on a plan going forward you could agree to meet up next week to see how things are progressing.

Discussion of Clinical Scenario 3

This is a difficult but very realistic discussion. There are two main strands to this scenario. One is to explore and manage the relative's understanding and expectations of Alzheimer's disease and secondly to address the issue of stem cell treatment she has read about.

- You need to show empathy throughout this scenario; this is particularly important as the relative is angry. By showing that you understand her concerns you will help to dispel some of the angry feeling she is experiencing.

- However angry the actor becomes you must stay calm and composed.

- Here you need to explore ICE in detail. The patient's daughter has ideas regarding what Alzheimer's entails but doesn't know much about the disease. Hence, this is an opportunity to explain the basics of the condition.

- She has concerns about who would provide any carers that her mum would need. This provides an opportunity to discuss the comprehensive multidisciplinary team assessment that her mum will undergo before discharge. It's an opportunity to reassure Mary as well that you won't send her mum home until it is safe to do so.

- Her expectations centre on the hope that a treatment she has read about in the paper might offer her mum some hope. It is perfectly reasonable for you to admit that you do not know much about the new stem cell treatment, but you should also say that you will find out more about it – perhaps by talking to your consultant.

- The challenge here is to manage these expectations.

- This is a perfect opportunity to talk about other sources of information available to the patient's daughter such as patient.co.uk, the NHS website and alzheimers.org.uk.

- Clearly it would be useful to meet with Mary at a later date to discuss how things are progressing so it would be great to arrange a follow up meeting.

Written Prioritisation Task – discussion

To reiterate – because of the very nature of this task there is no absolutely correct order in which you should put the options. Thus, the order illustrated below is not necessarily the order you may have chosen to rank these tasks. However, the points below represent some ideas of things you could consider. It is in no way exhaustive and represents a list of ideas rather than ideal answers. As discussed in *Chapter 5* it is crucial to provide a balance between justification and actions.

Order: E, C, D, B, A

> **E.** *"Your partner has sent you a text message asking you to call her as soon as possible"*
> - This is an important task as this may represent a personal or family emergency.
> - I would find it difficult to concentrate on other tasks if I didn't contact my partner straight away.
> - It would likely be a task that would take only a few minutes to complete.
> - I would contact her myself as it is not a task that I would be able to delegate to anyone else.
> - I would call her quickly and deal with the problem accordingly.

> **C.** *"A staff nurse informs you that the relative of a patient who has developed a postoperative complication wants to speak to you about making a formal complaint. The nurse informs you that the relative is very angry."*
> - I need to deal with this task early as it will play on my mind if left until later and this may also exacerbate the relative's anger.
> - It is important that patients and relatives are able to raise concerns and complaints.
> - I would ask the nurse to find out exactly what the relative was angry about so that I could begin to formulate a plan of how to handle the situation.
> - I would also ask the nurse to move the relative to the relatives' room.
> - I would ask the nurse to explain that I will be there shortly.
> - I would explore the relative's ideas, concerns and expectations and if they were still angry I would direct them to the local patient advice and liaison service (PALS) to facilitate their formal complaint.

D. *"A patient is due to have surgery this afternoon and has some questions"*
- This is a crucial task as it is important that the patient is fully informed before the procedure takes place.
- I would ask one of the nurses to establish what it was about the procedure that the patient wants to clarify so that I can formulate a plan as to what to say.
- If I felt it was going to be some time until I could do this task I would ask another member of my team to see if they might be able to help with this task.
- I would later reflect on how better to explain procedures to patients to avoid recurrence of these issues.

B. *"A health care assistant approaches you to discuss your registrar who she feels has been making derogatory comments about the care she is providing to patients"*
- This is an important issue as it may have an impact on the working of the team.
- It is important that all staff are able to work in a supportive environment.
- There are other more urgent clinical tasks which need completing first.
- Initially I would try to take responsibility for this task rather than delegate it.
- I would ask that we could meet together to discuss the issue further.
- If required I would involve the registrar in question and/or the consultant of the team in order to resolve the situation.

A. *"The ward clerk asks you to complete discharge summaries for four patients who were discharged yesterday"*
- It is crucial that GPs receive accurate and timely documentation regarding a patient's hospital admission, and discharge.
- There are other more urgent clinical tasks which need completing first.
- I would explain to the ward clerk that I have a few other issues to attend to first but I will deal with these discharges as soon as possible.
- Because of the other tasks I have to do I would first see if another member of my team (for example the FY1) was available to complete this task as it may be some time before I could complete it.
- I would reflect on why these tasks had been left until today to try to ensure that this did not happen again.

Reflection Section – discussion

Again, there are no absolute right and wrong answers in this section. Instead, you are being assessed on your ability to reflect on your decisions – you need to demonstrate that you have thought through your decisions clearly, and that you recognise that there is always room for improvement.

What aspect of this task did you find the hardest?
I found it difficult to know where to place option D ("A patient is due to have surgery this afternoon and has some questions"). The main reason for this was that it was difficult to know what exactly the patient wanted to find out. He may just have a simple question which would be very quick to answer or he may want a long conversation about his procedure, which could take a lot of time. It was therefore difficult to prioritise this task.

What did you do well?
I felt that I took responsibility for the tasks well. I did not shirk responsibility and tried to manage time to the best of my ability. Where I felt that the task was one that couldn't be delegated I took responsibility for the task and completed it myself.

What could you have done better?
I thought that I could've delegated more than I did. It is crucial to be able to work as part of a team and use people's skill sets appropriately. Therefore, on reflection, if I were to do this task again I would consider other members of the team who could help me with each task.

Appendix
Useful websites

Deanery Competition Ratios

http://gprecruitment.hee.nhs.uk/Recruitment/Competition-Ratios

It can be interesting to get an idea of how competitive each deanery has been over the last few years. However, it is important to note that while they give an indication of past competition, they cannot be used to predict future competition.

GMC's "Good Medical Practice"

http://www.gmc-uk.org/guidance/good_medical_practice.asp

This document is crucial reading for all doctors. It is particularly useful for those applying to GP training as it offers useful guidance on how to tackle common ethical scenarios.

GP National ST1 Personal Specification

http://specialtytraining.hee.nhs.uk/files/2014/09/2015-PS-GP-ST1-1-0.pdf

This document is a "must read" publication which is useful for both Stages 2 and 3 as it will help you focus on the areas against which you are being assessed.

Heath Protection Agency

https://www.gov.uk/government/organisations/public-health-england

This is a useful website which contains a wealth of information. It is particularly useful in refreshing knowledge of notifiable diseases and the like.

National Recruitment Office (NRO)

http://gprecruitment.hee.nhs.uk

The NRO website contains a plethora of useful resources and information. Particularly useful are links to each of the LETB deanery websites where you can find programme specific information and details.

NHS Foundation E-portfolio

https://www.nhseportfolios.org

Candidates who are current, or recent, FY2 doctors will have an e-portfolio. This can be helpful during Stage 1 when you are required to provide specific dates of hospital posts.

Oriel Application Portal

www.oriel.nhs.uk

Applications to GP specialty training are exclusively made through this website. The Oriel website offers an "Applicant User Guide" as well as a useful "frequently asked questions" section.

Pearson Vue

www.pearsonvue.co.uk

There is a useful tutorial available on the Pearson Vue website which takes you through the format of their online examinations.

Royal College of General Practitioners

www.rcgp.org.uk

The Royal College website will become very familiar to you during your time as a GP trainee. It has a wealth of information within it and is well worth a look.